Clinics in Human Lactation

How Breastfeeding Protects Women's Health Throughout the Lifespan:

The Psychoneuroimmunology of Human Lactation

Maureen Groer, RN, Ph.D., FAAN

Kathleen Kendall-Tackett, Ph.D., IBCLC, FAPA

Hale Publishing, L.P.

How Breastfeeding Protects Women's Health Throughout the Lifespan:

The Psychoneuroimmunology of Human Lactation

Maureen Groer, RN, Ph.D., FAAN

Kathleen Kendall-Tackett, Ph.D., IBCLC, FAPA

Hale Publishing, L.P.

1712 N. Forest St.

Amarillo, TX 79106-7017

806-376-9900

800-378-1317

www.iBreastfeeding.com

www.halepublishing.com

Library of Congress Control Number: 2011925700

ISBN-13: 978-0-9833075-4-9

Printing and Binding: Malloy, Inc.

Contents

Introduction. Why Would Breastfeeding Protect Maternal Health?

Over the past decade, researchers have discovered that breastfeeding is more protective of maternal health than was previously imagined, and that it dramatically lowers women's risk of disease throughout their lives. In particular, researchers have documented the impact of breastfeeding on the risk of cardiovascular disease, metabolic syndrome, and diabetes during middle and old age. Since these conditions are common causes of premature mortality for women, these findings are of particular interest.

For example, a study of 139,681 postmenopausal women found that a lifetime history of lactation of more than 12 months related to lower rates of hypertension, diabetes, hyperlipidemia, and cardiovascular disease (Schwarz et al., 2009). The mean age of the women in the study was 63. Similarly, the CARDIA study included 704 women enrolled during their first pregnancy and followed them for 20 years (Gunderson et al., 2010). Women without gestational diabetes who had breastfed for at least one month had a 56% reduced risk for metabolic syndrome, and there was an 86% reduction in risk for women with gestational diabetes.

A cohort analysis of 2,516 parous, midlife women who participated in the SWAN study found that breastfeeding duration lowered prevalence of metabolic syndrome in a dose-response way (Ram et al., 2008). Specifically, the longer they breastfed, the lower the risk. Duration of lactation inversely correlated with a number of risk factors for cardiovascular disease, such as current body mass index (BMI), waist circumference, blood pressure, fasting glucose, insulin, triglycerides, and total and LDL cholesterol.

Longer duration of lactation reduced risk of type-2 diabetes in phases I and II of the Nurses' Health Study (N=85,585 and 73,418 parous women; Stuebe, Rich-Edwards, Willett, Manson, & Michels, 2005). The mean age of participants was 50 years. The researchers found that each additional year of lactation decreased risk of metabolic syndrome by 15%. This effect was independent of BMI, diet, exercise, or smoking. Exclusive breastfeeding associated with greatest reduction in risk and a longer duration per pregnancy resulted in the greatest long-term reduction in risk (e.g., risk was lower if a woman breastfed one baby for 12 months vs. two babies for six months each). The authors concluded that sustained lactation-associated metabolic changes may have profound effects on diabetes risk.

The sum of these research findings raises an intriguing question: why would breastfeeding have these long-term effects on maternal health? It is a question we believe we can answer by drawing upon the research in a field known as psychoneuroimmunology (PNI). Psychoneuroimmunology is an emerging, interdisciplinary science in which there is consideration of ways in which the human mind and immune system interact and influence each other. Over the past nearly 40 years, a body of evidence clearly shows that stress and coping may produce changes in immunity. These changes, in turn, can result in health effects that contribute to disease.

Typically, scientists in PNI analyze changes in immune cells, such as lymphocytes, macrophages, and Natural Killer cells, and immune secretions, such as immunoglobulins, cytokines, and chemokines. These are usually measured in peripheral blood, in cultures of cells, or in mucosal secretions, such as saliva. Human milk contains cells, cytokines, and immunoglobulins, along with many, many other immunomodulating chemicals. Little is known about how these factors are regulated in human milk. Emerging evidence suggests that maternal factors, such as stress, fatigue, and depression, could potentially produce immunological changes in milk and, under extreme circumstances, could potentially affect milk output. It is also being appreciated that the lactational postpartum state is truly unique behaviorally and physiologically, designed by nature to allow the mother to optimally nurture and feed her newborn infant. Supporting this state is a responsibility of healthcare providers, families, and even governments to ensure the healthy outcomes of the nursing infant.

Previously, the health "benefits of breastfeeding" were largely considered to be confined to infancy, and were focused on infant benefits. Now, much new data have suggested that breastfeeding has longer-term, even life-long, effects for both the mother and the nursing infant. Some of these benefits may be conferred through immunological and endocrine programming that occurs early in life.

Clearly, new knowledge about human milk and lactation is of interest to maternal-child healthcare science and practice. The new concepts that breastfeeding and human milk might confer benefits to immune, neurological, and metabolic processes that ultimately translate into protection from adult diseases now bears scrutiny through the life span. This monograph will provide the latest evidence on how breastfeeding and human milk are the biological norms for mother and baby, and how artificial feeding puts both of them at risk for health problems throughout their lives. Note that we consider several phenomena here: the actual maternal-infant breastfeeding relationship, the unique psychobiology of the lactational state, and the biology of human milk. The three can be considered separately, as well as together. A modern practice by today's busy professional woman is to provide human milk to her infant through pumping, often for many months, as the sole source of nutrition. While this is clearly preferable to artificial-milk feeding, what is missing is the intimate skin-to-skin psychobiology of the physical act of breastfeeding, which in and of itself may confer PNI benefits.

This monograph will present information on the science of PNI and apply it to the maternal-infant breastfeeding dyad, presenting the latest evidence that will inform practice and, we hope, ultimately policy.

Chapter 1. Breast Differentiation, Lactogenesis, and Lactation: Basic Concepts

Breast Development

Breast development primarily occurs after the onset of puberty, when ovarian steroids, estrogen and progesterone, begin to be cyclically secreted by the ovaries under the influences of pituitary stimulating hormones. The post-pubertal development of the breast takes around four years, and no further development occurs after the age of about 16 years until pregnancy and lactation (http://mammary.nih.gov/reviews/development/Human-breast001/index.html).

The human female breast undergoes its final differentiation during lactation, and thus, if a woman never lactates, the final developmental maturation of the breast is arrested. Women who breastfeed are somewhat protected from the later development of breast cancer, and in part, this is thought to be due to the lack of full differentiation of the breasts when women do not lactate. A study of Chinese women found a reduced breast cancer risk in women who breastfed. Breastfeeding for more than 24 months per child produced an odds ratio of 0.46 when compared to women who breastfed each child for one to six months. The more months a woman breastfed in her reproductive years, the greater was her protection from breast cancer (Zheng et al., 2000).

In studies of American women, the effect has also been found, although the size of the protective effect varies from study to study. In a study of both White and Black women from North Carolina, any breastfeeding at all was associated with a slight reduction in breast cancer incidence (Hall, Moorman, Millikan, & Newman, 2005). American women who have their first pregnancy after the age of 25 years have an increased risk of breast cancer, but this risk is reduced by breastfeeding for cancers that are estrogen dependent (Ma, Bernstein, Ross, & Ursin, 2006).

The physiological mechanism through which lactation affords breast cancer protection is unknown. Part of the protection is parity itself, as nulliparous women are more at risk for postmenopausal breast cancer than parous women. Mammary stem cells are constantly being renewed through breast development and maturation, and one concept is that the breasts of women who become pregnant and lactate contain more differentiated epithelial stem cells than nulliparous women (Russo et al., 2006). Normally, mammary stem cells occupy a niche in the breast tissue which is closely regulated, and loss of this regulation might lead to malignant transformation.

Interestingly, there is at least one compound in human milk that has been identified in vitro as anti-tumorigenic. HAMLET (human alpha-lactalbumin made lethal to tumor cells) has been identified and characterized by Swedish researcher, Catharina Svanborg. It is a molecular complex in human milk that kills tumor cells by an apoptotic-like process, and it has been shown to kill mouse mammary cell lines (Pettersson-Kastberg et al., 2009). This compound is also currently being tested for antibacterial properties against *S. Pneumoniae* through a Gates Foundation grant to Hazeline Hakansson at the University of Buffalo (http://www.acsu.buffalo.edu/~andersh/research/HAMLET.asp).

Breast development occurs during puberty under the influence of estrogen, then moves into a further stage of differentiation in pregnancy, stimulated by progesterone, prolactin, and placental lactogen (Neville & Morton, 2001). This maturation involves the terminal duct lobular units, which arise from the breast milk ducts. Milk synthesis is stimulated by these developments during the second trimester of pregnancy, and the mammary cells begin to produce many milk proteins. Some women may notice a small amount of milk secretion occurring during pregnancy, and by late pregnancy, 30 mLs/day of colostrum can be produced (Cox, Kent, Casey, Owens, & Hartmann, 1999). Extensive tissue remodeling and vascularization prepares the breast tissue during pregnancy, influenced by the cytokine, vascular endothelial growth factor (VEGF; Qiu et al., 2008). Lipid also accumulates in the mammary cells, and the breasts undergo a stage of differentiation that is termed Lactogenesis I. During Lactogenesis I, the tight junctions between adjacent glandular epithelial cells in the alveoli are open and permeable. When lactation becomes fully established these tight junctions close and are impermeable, thus allowing milk to be stored in the alveoli (Nguyen & Neville, 1998). Thus the constituents of milk produced during Lactogenesis I consists of immunoglobulins, many large proteins, and bacteriostatic oligosaccharide molecules, as well as a filtrate containing water and electrolytes. The key event that marks the termination of Lactogenesis I is the closure of the epithelial tight junctions of the alveolar epithelium, which then inhibits the filtration of water, large molecules, and sodium into the milk. Normally, these junctions remain closed throughout the remainder of lactation.

Lactogenesis II is marked by the secretion of large amounts of milk following birth, due in part to the drop in progesterone at birth (Neville & Morton, 2001). This milk is lower in sodium and chloride and higher in lactose. A fall in progesterone is a prerequisite for development of Lactogenesis II. Both estrogen and progesterone fall dramatically at birth and remain lower in lactating compared to non-lactating mothers. Other endocrine requirements for Lactogenesis II include cortisol, thyroid hormone, prolactin, and insulin. Normally, this stage occurs around three to four days after birth, as long as the infant is suckling and prolactin levels are high. The final stage of lactation is Lactogenesis III. Lactogenesis III is thought to be largely due to autocrine influence within the breasts themselves, so that milk production is dependent upon demand by the infant.

Physiological Influence on Lactation

There are many physiological influences that promote lactogenesis and successful lactation in human females. The unique endocrine milieu present right after birth provides the background for successful lactation. At birth the pregnancy levels of estrogen and progesterone fall, while prolactin and oxytocin secretion rise in response to suckling. Prolactin is produced by the adenohypophysis (anterior pituitary gland) and released into the bloodstream where it can reach its many target receptors. These receptors are in the breast, as well as on many different types of cells throughout the body. Prolactin is released under the influence of the dopaminergic system, with dopamine inhibiting its release from the pituitary. It had been previously believed that prolactin was not influenced by a releasing factor, a pathway known to be an important regulator for the synthesis and release of other pituitary hormones. While a prolactin-releasing peptide has been identified and is known to influence prolactin secretion in tissue culture, its role in human lactation has not yet been established (Sun, Fujiwara, Adachi, & Inoue, 2005). In the past, lactation was inhibited by giving new mothers the drug, Bromocriptine, which stimulates dopamine production in the brain, thus inhibiting prolactin release. Interestingly, when Bromocriptine was administered to lactating hamster dams, it caused them to have disturbed maternal behavior and even injure and kill their pups (McCarthy, Curran, & Siegel, 1994).

There are prolactin receptors in the human breast, and prolactin binds to these receptors to stimulate the human breast to produce milk. Once bound, prolactin stimulates synthesis of mRNA of milk proteins. The infant's latch and suckling is the trigger for release of prolactin from the anterior pituitary, and several minutes of sucking are required for prolactin release.

At Lactogenesis II, milk volume reaches about 500 mL per day. The milk itself also changes from birth through the production of first, transitional, and then mature milk. Both the nutritional and immunological nature of the milk changes. Lactogenesis II is a critical stage for lactational success. In many animal species, including humans, obesity impairs Lactogenesis II, partially through impairment of prolactin release in response to suckling (Rasmussen & Kjolhede, 2004).

Factors that Influence Breastfeeding Success

Breastfeeding success is affected by many additional factors. The earlier there is successful latch and feeding, the more likely it is that breastfeeding will be a long-term success for mother and baby. The first hours after birth and the first week of lactation are critical to long-term breastfeeding, and the most frequent problems are delayed onset of Lactogenesis II, poor latch, and infant feeding difficulties due to labor medications. Factors that are known to impair Lactogenesis II include obesity, primiparity (especially if the infant is large), maternal diabetes, and labor stress (Dewey, Nommsen-Rivers, Heinig, & Cohen, 2003). Infant feeding problems can be the result of flat or inverted nipples, poor latch, use of supplemental feedings, and pacifier use. Labor stress is often the result of a prolonged labor experience (Dewey et al., 2003). Preterm delivery and exposure of the mother during pregnancy to steroids is also known to impair lactation (Rasmussen & Kjolhede, 2004).

The infant and mother have the opportunity to begin their lifelong intimate relationship in the delivery room. It is here that breastfeeding should be first initiated. This is most optimal when neither the infant nor the mother is affected by medications that could impair alertness. Usually less than 5 mLs of colostrum is produced in that first feeding, but successful latch is important. The infant has "practiced" primitive neonatal reflexes involved in rooting, sucking, and swallowing, and at term is born with these reflex capacities to initiate feeding almost immediately (Colson, Meek, & Hawdon, 2008).

Early skin-to-skin contact between the mother and her infant promotes these reflexes, and other reflex responses have also been noted with skin-to-skin contact. Early research suggested that uninterrupted skin-to-skin contact immediately after birth was a key factor in successful breastfeeding (Righard & Alade, 1990). This contact allowed for the emergence of other primitive neonatal reflexes. In a study of nine full-term infants receiving "kangaroo" or skin-to-skin contact within one minute of birth, and continuing until successful latch and breastfeeding had been initiated, eight infants "crawled" to the mother's breast and successfully latched within 74 minutes post birth. This activity had the added benefit of distracting mothers from the discomfort of episiotomy or laceration repair (Walters, Boggs, Ludington-Hoe, Price, & Morrison, 2007).

Once the mother-infant dyad has been moved from the labor and delivery suite to the postpartum unit, breastfeeding success is aided by the practice of rooming-in. Here the mother has the opportunity to begin to interpret and understand her infant's cues and respond. Postpartum units are often very busy places, and mothers may be interrupted many times during their stays. Most startling is the data from Case Western University researchers (Morrison, Ludington-Hoe, & Anderson, 2006) reporting that breastfeeding mothers were interrupted 54 times per day, with most interruptions being less than or equal to nine minutes. These interruptions included visits to the patient's room and telephone calls. Such interference with the establishment of the maternal-infant dyadic relationship is bound to affect breastfeeding success in the hospital.

Maturity of the suck and swallow mechanisms is also essential for successful infant breastfeeding (Udall, 2007). The development of the anatomical and physiological processes that are required for latching, sucking, and swallowing begin early in gestation. At around 18 to 20 weeks of gestation, the fetus makes sucking movements. Towards the end of pregnancy, the fetus actually regularly swallows about 500 mL of amniotic fluid a day. However, premature and small for gestational age infants are at risk for difficulty with coordination of the latch, and suck and swallow mechanisms. Very low birthweight infants are often not only unable to breastfeed, but lack the maturity of the gastrointestinal tract. New evidence suggests that preterm mothers' colostrum and milk may be particularly developmentally programmed to meet the needs of these small infants.

Composition of Milk

Milk is secreted continuously in the breast cells known as lactocytes. The lactocytes line the alveoli, with capillaries in close apposition to the alveoli that supply the lactocytes with the building blocks of the various nutritional and immunological components of milk. The lactocytes assemble the molecules in milk and secrete these molecules in the fluid milk matrix through the lactocyte membrane into the alveolus. Table 1-1 lists the major components of human milk (Jensen, 1995).

Table 1-1. Components of Human Milk

Immune Components	Secretory Immunoglobulin A
	Lactoferrin
	Lysozyme
	Cytokines and chemokines
	Growth factors
Nutritional	67 kcal/100 mL
	DHA and ARA
	Carnitine
	Calories
	Lipids, carbohydrates and proteins
	Oligosaccharides
	Vitamins
	Minerals
	Hormones
	Enzymes
Cells	Macrophages
	Lymphocytes
	Natural Killer cells
	Epithelial cells

Milk synthesis and release is a complex process that involves many physiological systems. One pathway is by exocytosis, in which components, such as proteins and lactose, are released through the cell membrane in Golgi system secretory vesicles. The fat in milk is present as globules which are produced in the cytoplasm from intracellular lipid. There is also a direct pathway for water, ions, and glucose through the cell membrane. Finally, a pathway between adjacent cells, the paracellular pathway, allows plasma proteins and cells to traverse between the blood stream and milk.

Interestingly, the composition of milk varies significantly between species, and within species, changes over the course of time. Thus, colostrum is a vastly different secretion compared to mature milk, and milk from preterm mothers is qualitatively different from term milk. There are three stages of milk synthesis in sequence in the lactating female: colostrum, transitional milk, and mature milk. Colostrum is thick and yellow, and has high concentrations of cells, immunoglobulins, lysozyme, and lactoferrin, as well as electrolytes, such as sodium and chloride, and low concentrations of casein, lactose, potassium, citrate, calcium, and phosphate. Typically, colostrum is secreted for about three days, and then transitional milk is produced for about seven to ten days. Transitional milk is creamier in appearance than colostrum and contains less protein, but higher concentrations of lactose, fat, calories, and vitamins. Mature milk is then produced throughout the rest of the time a mother lactates. If a mother experiences difficulties in early lactation, the composition of the milk will sometimes reflect lack of maturation of Lactogenesis.

In general, human milk is highly anti-inflammatory and contains a system of molecules and cells that protect the immature infant gut from inflammation, while allowing the establishment of the normal microbiotic flora that is necessary to inhibit pathogenic bacteria from flourishing and invading. The infant is essentially born sterile, and within hours has accumulated a huge number of microorganisms from its exposure to the vagina and perineum of the mother, the colostrum it has ingested, her skin and mucosa, and the surrounding environment. While the human infant's gut may be hypersensitive to inflammatory signal, milk contains multiple molecules that oppose inflammation. These include inflammatory cytokine receptors, glycans, fatty acids, adiponectin, anti-inflammatory cytokines, such as IL-10, along with multiple other factors. The more immature preterm infant's gut is even more susceptible to inflammation, and if not provided human milk, the preterm infant is far more at risk for necrotizing enterocolitis (Israel, 1994; Kliegman, Walker, & Yolken, 1993).

Cells in Milk

Colostrum contains the highest percentage of white blood cells, but some cells can be found in milk throughout lactation. The majority of colostral cells are macrophages (40-60%), neutrophils, along with lymphocytes, and epithelial cells. There is considerable evidence that these cells are not mere incidental passengers in milk, but rather have critically important roles in protecting the infant. The cells are alive, secreting cytokines, and capable of cell-cell interaction with each other and intestinal luminal cells. They appear to have a role in defense of the infant with regard to microbial pathogens. Macrophages are antigen-processing and phagocytic cells. When milk has transitioned to the mature milk stage, there are 80-90% macrophages present, at a concentration of 104-105 human milk macrophages per mL. The cells in milk are hardy and have been shown to survive for as long as a week in baboons and lambs. The T cells in milk appear not to be naïve cells, but rather effector memory T cells (Sabbaj et al., 2005). In fact, milk appears enriched with these cells, present at higher concentration than in the peripheral blood.

Immune Components of Milk

Milk contains multiple components that are immunomodulatory. Well known for many years is the protective secretory IgA in human milk. However, many other molecules with immune function or effect are present in milk. These molecules may protect the infant from infection, modulate the gastrointestinal maturation and function, and impact the development of the infant's immune system. Lactoferrin and lysozyme have been well described as antimicrobial proteins in milk. Lactoferrin in milk appears to promote the recruitment of leukocytes and activation of dendritic cells (de la Rosa, Yang, Tewary, Varadhachary, & Oppenheim, 2008). This may foster activation of milk cells and enhancement of immunological function within the milk and intestines of the infant.

There are also many cytokines in human milk that appear to be active in the infant gut. Our lab has measured many of these cytokines through a technique called multiplexing. Using an instrument (the Luminex-200), we are able to use antibody-coated beads and fluorescent dyes to produce a fluorescence unique for each cytokine and measure many cytokines at once in a tiny volume of milk (25 ul). We have found that cytokines, chemokines, and growth factors cluster together in unique ways that may inform our future studies about origins and functions of the many cytokines in milk (Groer & Beckstead, 2011).

Immunoglobulins in Milk

The major immunoglobulin in human milk is secretory Immunoglobulin A (SIgA), although smaller amounts of other Igs are present. A remarkable mechanism exists for producing SIgA in both adequate amounts and with finely tuned specificity. SIgA is produced in enormous amounts (12 g/L) in colostrum, and even in mature milk 1 g/L is routinely produced (Newburg & Walker, 2007). Figure 1-1 depicts the pathways through which maternal antigen exposure ultimately produces Igs in milk.

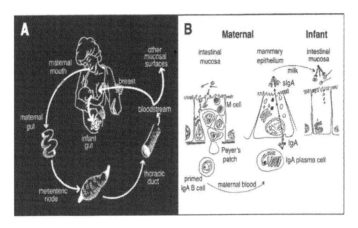

Figure 1-1. Pathways through which maternal antigen exposure produces Igs in milk. From Newburg & Walker, 2007. Used with permission.

IgA is synthesized by plasma cells that have migrated and homed to the lactating breast. There are links between the maternal gastrointestinal and respiratory tracts that allow the mother's B cells to secrete the specific antigens to which she has been exposed. Known as the entero- and broncho-mammeric links, the processes begin by the dendritic cells capturing antigenic material and presenting antigen to T cells, which then activate B cells with the capability of synthesizing Igs to the antigen. These B cells migrate from this initial site of activation, which could be gut-associated lymphoid tissue (GALT) or bronchial-associated lymphoid tissue (BALT), to other areas. These cells may express homing receptors, and they seek the mammary epithelium. Once in the breast, they secrete immunoglobulins on the basolateral membrane of the mammary epithelial cells. A receptor is present for the IgA to attach, known as the polyimmunoglobulin receptor, and the entire complex passes through the epithelial cells and is enzymatically altered so that it becomes secretory IgA.

SIgA in milk is a dimer and is highly resistant to digestive enzymes and acid, and, therefore, is active in the infant's intestinal lumen. The SIgA in the intestine binds by the secretory component to the intestinal epithelium, forming a large surface area of antisepsis. Antigens that find their way into the intestine are then confronted by antibody which binds and essentially removes the antigen from having a deleterious effect. The intestinal epithelium is thus protected, and the antigen cannot enter into the infant's circulation through transintestinal passages. Pathogens represent a potential threat to the nursing infant, but that threat is largely mitigated by the specific SIgAs that are synthesized by these cells that have been activated and "alerted" by exposure to the antigens in the mother's gastrointestinal and respiratory tracts. The pathogens that an infant is exposed to are from the most proximate caregiver, and that is usually the nursing mother. Nature has designed a mechanism that allows a mother to protect her infant from her own resident potentially harmful pathogens.

There is a possibility that this mechanism is even more finely orchestrated than what has just been described. Recently, the protective effect of breastfeeding on Respiratory Syncytial Virus (RSV) bronchiolitis in infants was described as a process in which the immunomodulatory constituents of human milk differed in breastfeeding mothers of infants with bronchiolitis compared to milk from mothers with well infants (Bryan, Hart, Forsyth, & Gibson, 2007). There were more viable immune cells in this milk, and the cells, when stimulated, produced a skewed Th2 (humoral) cytokine pattern in response to stimulation with RSV. Studies such as this suggest that there may be subtle biochemical messages that are transmitted from mother to infant, and vice versa, possibly "danger" signals, allowing for the possibility of specific and differential responses on both parts to these danger signals. In line with that reasoning, the study by our lab (Groer & Shelton, 2009) found that postpartum breastfeeding mothers who were heavy, vigorous exercisers in the early postpartum produced a different profile of cytokines in their milk as compared to non- or light-exercising postpartum mothers. The cytokines in the milk were skewed toward a proinflammatory profile, but the SIgA was not altered.

In another study of milk from mothers with pre-eclampsia, it was found that proinflammatory cytokines, such as IL-8 and TNF-α, were in higher concentration (Erbagci et al., 2005). This was suggested to be "biological information" to the infant about maternal health. Another study of diabetic and hypothyroid mothers found that milk volume was lower in these groups (Miyake, Tahara, Koike, & Tanizawa, 1989). It is also well known that obese women have delayed lactogenesis and shortened length of time of breastfeeding (Jevitt, Hernandez, & Groer, 2007). It is possible that stress associated with these illnesses or conditions, medications administered, or metabolic pathophysiological changes could potentially alter milk composition and functional ability.

A new frontier of investigation relates to the possible influence of multiple maternal factors on immunological components of human milk. The next two chapters will explore these biobehavioral pathways, hormones, neuroendocrine secretions, and immune messenger molecules.

Chapter 2. Basic Overview of the Human Stress Response

Stress is a term commonly used in everyday discourse. The technical definition of stress is when the demands in the environment exceed a person's ability to cope. There are many examples of stressors that can include issues with family, job, or other relationships; a history of abuse or trauma; losing a job; or losing a loved one. Stress is studied a number of different ways. Researchers might measure the stressor itself, how the person reacts to it, or long-term consequences of exposure to stressful events.

When we perceive any type of threat, our bodies mobilize our internal forces in order to deal with the threat. The brain activates two primary outflow pathways: the sympathetic system and the hypothalamic-pituitary-adrenal (HPA) axis. Both of these activate the immune and inflammatory systems. Generally speaking, the stress response is adaptive and designed to preserve our lives, but it is meant to be an acute response. When it is acute, it increases immune cells to the site of challenge. Problems arise when the stress response is chronically activated. Chronic stress is often harmful and increases the risk of disease, including infections, inflammatory diseases, and autoimmune diseases.

Sympathetic Adrenomedullary System (SAM) and Parasympathetic System

The first system the body activates when faced with an acute threat is the SAM, producing the "fight or flight" response. Stressors are first perceived in the limbic system, which sends signals through the sympathetic and parasympathetic systems. These systems generally act to oppose each other. The sympathetic system sends impulses to the adrenal medulla, which releases epinephrine and norepinephrine. Epinephrine and norepinephrine, the catecholamines, increase cardiac output by elevating heart rate and stroke volume. These stress hormones also redistribute immune cells so that they can easily reach a site of injury, and they mobilize fuel sources. Catecholamines work through the central nervous system to increase alertness and arousal. Generally speaking, SAM is activated only in times of acute stress, but it can be tonically active in some individuals. These individuals might also be highly reactive to minor perturbations.

The parasympathetic arm of the autonomic nervous system opposes SAM through activation of the vagal nerve. This may act to regulate allostatic load (Thayer & Sternberg, 2006). Allostasis is the body's attempt to adapt to the changing environment and respond to chronic stress. When the amount of stress overwhelms the system, allostatic load occurs, resulting in "wear and tear" on the body's systems, which may contribute to the pathophysiological process involved in a variety of chronic illnesses. When vagal function decreases, fasting glucose elevates, and proinflammatory cytokines, acute-phase proteins, and cortisol increases–all of which constitute allostatic load.

The HPA Axis

In response to stress, SAM and the HPA axis are activated at the same time by the limbic system. The HPA axis is more gradual in its effects. In response to a threat, the HPA axis activates a hormonal cascade initiated by release of corticotrophin-releasing hormone (CRH) from the hypothalamus, which stimulates the pituitary to release adrenocorticotrophic hormone (ACTH). ACTH then circulates in the blood and acts on adrenal cortical cells, causing the release of glucocorticoids (GCs; Maes et al., 2009). Cortisol plays an important role in our survival. In times of stress, cortisol increases fuel available for the body by increasing food intake and causing glucose to be available as a fuel. It also suppresses other functions not immediately essential, such as reproduction (Landys, Ramenofsky, & Wingfield, 2006). Cortisol also enhances the effects of the SAM on cardiovascular function during stress (McEwen, 2003).

Cortisol suppresses the immune system and is anti-inflammatory. It downregulates the inflammatory and immune responses and keeps them within safe limits. Cortisol decreases inflammation by binding to receptors on immune cells, which is thought to account, in part, for its immunosuppressive effects (Adcock, Ito, & Barnes, 2004).

Cortisol levels are often abnormally low in depressed people. They may also be cortisol-resistant, meaning they are less sensitive to existing cortisol. In either case, cortisol fails to restrain the inflammatory response (Dhabhar & McEwen, 2001). Pace and colleagues (2007) noted that cortisol resistance occurs in up to 80% of depressed patients, and has been one of the most reproducible biologic symptoms of depression. Chronic exposure to inflammatory cytokines, from either medical illness or chronic stress, could impair receptor function, which may result in glucocorticoid resistance.

When cortisol is not functioning effectively, there is nothing to curb inflammation, which could lead to severe and continuous tissue damage. However, too much cortisol over a longer term can also contribute to allostatic load, and thus to disease. A dysregulated HPA axis is potentially an early indicator of allostasis and can manifest in cortisol levels that are either too high or too low, unusual patterns in the early-morning-awakening rise in cortisol, abnormalities in the dexamethasone suppression test, and flattened cortisol rhythms across the day (McEwen, 2003). A number of conditions or situations result in a chronically activated HPA. These include melancholic depression, anorexia nervosa, obsessive-compulsive disorder, panic anxiety, alcoholism, alcohol and narcotic withdrawal, excessive exercising, poorly controlled diabetes mellitus, hyperthyroidism, and childhood sexual abuse (Tsigos & Chrousos, 2002).

Cortisol levels also change depending on time of day, season, and reproductive state. For example, cortisol levels rise upon awakening, and this allows us to go about our activities of daily living (Wust, Federenko, Hellhammer, & Kirschbaum, 2000). In fact, getting out of bed in the morning requires both cortisol and the SAM in order to ensure adequate blood flow to the brain and to mobilize metabolic fuels for the energy needs of the day. Interestingly, people are more likely to have a heart attack in the morning, particularly Monday morning, because of the morning rise in blood pressure and heart rate (Giles, 2005). The normal daily rhythm of cortisol, and our ability to produce cortisol in response to stressors are healthy phenomena. But cortisol is meant for an acute response. Prolonged exposure and levels that are too high or too low can cause physical damage and are considered maladaptive (the so-called U-shaped curve; Gunnar & Quevedo, 2007).

People experiencing chronic stress can also have too little cortisol (known as hypocortisolemia). Some conditions where hypocortisolemia are likely to occur include atypical depression with exhaustion (Gold, Goodman, & Chrousos, 1988), posttraumatic stress disorder (PTSD; Yehuda, 1997), addiction disorders (Schuder, 2005), fibromyalgia (McBeth et al., 2005), and postpartum depression (Groer & Morgan, 2007). Cortisol levels can also be low in combat veterans with PTSD, who may have lower morning cortisol (Boscarino, 1996) and lower 24-hour cortisol levels than normal values of men without PTSD (Yehuda, 1997).

Inflammatory Cytokines and Acute-Phase Reactants

The immune system also responds to stress by increasing levels of inflammation. Inflammation is usually provoked by pathogen associated molecular patterns (PAMPS), which bind to toll-like receptors (TLRs) on the membranes of immune cells (Beutler, 2004). Neurotransmitters and neuropeptides can also activate inflammatory cells (Sternberg, 2006), as can "danger signals," such as complement, heat shock proteins, and other products of injured or dying cells (Matzinger, 2002). Norepinephrine may also increase stress-induced proinflammatory cytokines within central nervous system and peripheral circulation (Blandino, Barnum, & Deak, 2006; Johnson et al., 2005). Sympathetic fibers innervate virtually every immune organ, but the density and distribution of innervation varies between organs. Further, immune cells have receptors for stress hormones or neurotransmitters, which means that stress exerts regulatory control over immune function. A stress-induced autonomic-inflammatory reflex may explain how stress is involved in metabolic, vascular, and autoimmune diseases (Bierhaus, Humpert, & Nawroth, 2006).

As described earlier, inflammation can cause tissue damage if not controlled. To prevent this from occurring, our body's anti-inflammatory processes normally contain inflammation. These anti-inflammatory molecules include cortisol and anti-inflammatory cytokines, such as interleukin-10 (IL-10) and transforming growth factor-beta (TGF-ß). The inflammatory response, if inappropriate, excessive, or long-lasting, becomes the underpinnings of many human diseases, such as coronary heart disease (CHD).

Many cell types, including macrophages, endothelium, fat cells, muscle cells, and liver, release inflammatory cytokines in response to danger signals. Proinflammatory cytokines, such as interleukin-1 (IL-1), IL-6, and tumor necrosis factor-α (TNF-α), act to provoke inflammatory changes locally and on distant systems, such as the brain and liver.

IL-6 is one of the most important primary mediators of allostasis. It leads to the acute-phase inflammatory response and controls the hepatic acute-phase response. It is an endogenous proinflammatory cytokine produced by adipose tissue, macrophages, adipocytes, T-cells, and endothelium. IL-6 stimulates sickness behaviors, fever, fatigue, hematopoiesis, and immune responses. IL-6 has been correlated with measures of CHD and insulin resistance and is higher in obese individuals (Brunn et al., 2003).

When exposed to IL-6, liver cells augment expression of acute-phase proteins, including fibrinogen and C-reactive protein (CRP). CRP is released in response to acute injury, infection, or other inflammatory stimuli, such as inflammatory diseases, necrosis, and trauma (Wilson, Ryan, & Boyle, 2006). CRP is a marker of low-grade inflammation that is largely produced in the liver. High levels of CRP have been associated with obesity, insulin resistance, and an increased risk of type-2 diabetes (Kip et al., 2004; Lakka et al., 2005; Wilson et al., 2006). CRP is also a useful marker of allostatic load, and it predicts cardiovascular risk. Adding CRP to a global risk prediction model improved cardiovascular risk classification in participants in the Women's Health Study, particularly for those with a ten year risk of 5% to 20% (Cook, Buring, & Ridker, 2006). High BMI showed stronger associations with CRP than physical activity (Mora, Lee, Buring, & Ridker, 2006).

Bidirectional Communication between Brain and Immune System

The CNS and immune system communicate with each other in a bidirectional fashion. For example, the immune system alters the functioning of the CNS through the release of proinflammatory cytokines (Dantzer & Kelley, 2007; Maier & Watkins, 1998). The CNS and immune system release regulatory proteins, such as cytokines. Cytokines can influence central nervous system function and behavior, and also act as intercellular messengers to alter inflammation and immunity (Maier & Watkins, 1998; Watkins & Maier, 2000). For example, when there is an immune challenge or stress exposure, proinflammatory cytokine expression increases in the brain and in the periphery. Many types of stressors increase circulating and central levels of proinflammatory cytokines, such as interleukin-1ß (IL-1ß) and interleukin-6 (IL-6; Huang, Takaki, & Arimura, 1997; LeMay, Otterness, Vander, & Luger, 1990; LeMay, Vander, & Kluger, 1990; Maes, 2001; Shizuya et al., 1997, 1998; Steptoe, Willemsen, Owen, Flower, & Mohamed-Ali, 2001).

Proinflammatory cytokines, such as IL-1ß and IL-6, can regulate the stress response by binding to receptors that can activate the HPA axis (Bethin Vogt, & Muglia, 2000). In addition, proinflammatory cytokines mediate the sickness syndrome observed following both infection and stress (Bluthe, Michaud, Poli, & Dantzer, 2000; Dantzer & Kelley, 2007; Maier & Watkins, 1998; Watkins & Maier, 2000). Sickness syndrome conserves metabolic resources during periods of challenge, and includes loss of appetite and consequent weight loss, decreased activity, loss of interest in pleasurable activities (anhedonia), and enhanced pain sensitivity (hyperalgesia and allodynia).

Is There Stress in the Postpartum?

While for most parents there is joy and satisfaction with the birth of a baby, many situations or events occurring in the postpartum period are stressors with potential for taxing patterns of function. The evolution of our understanding of postpartum stressors parallels that of the understanding of the construct of stress itself. Early reports focusing on stressors as major life events were followed by attempts to identify more specific stressors or effects of smaller everyday adverse events. More recent reports center on appraisal or perception of stress as the crucial variable. Whatever the source, it is postulated that the stress response follows appraisal of the event or situation as stressful. Thus, a stressor initiates a response, but the stress response is mediated by perception of stress.

The stressors that face both breast and formula feeding mothers can be categorized very generally as physical, intrapersonal, and interpersonal. As we shall see later in this monograph, postpartum mothers appear to have an ability to screen out a lot of the minor stressful events that might ordinarily perturb or bother them. Nevertheless, there is some degree of stress for all new mothers and fathers. Our research group analyzed data from a cross sectional study of postpartum mothers measured between four and six weeks after the birth of the baby. In an analysis of 167 narratives, mothers reported a variety of things that they would describe as the most stressful event. Four salient themes emerged from analysis of all 167 stressful events: 1) Stressors Within the Mother-Newborn Dyad, 2) Role Strain, 3) Stressors External to the Mother-Newborn Dyad, and 4) Lack of Support. Stressors within the Maternal-Newborn Dyad was the predominant theme, containing 42% of the total responses, including stressors such as children's health problems, lack of sleep, newborn crying, and breastfeeding problems. Stress related to breastfeeding was reported by only seven women (4%), even though almost half of the 167 mothers who reported on stress were breastfeeding their newborns. In fact, breastfeeding may act as a kind of buffer for mothers between the stressor, the appraisal, and the response.

Summary

Stress has a direct biological effect on disease risk and includes responses by the sympathetic nervous system, HPA axis, and inflammatory response system. Communication between the brain and immune system is bidirectional. Stress causes the brain to trigger the immune response, and the immune response can induce changes in the central nervous system, resulting in a constellation of behaviors known as sickness syndrome. Chronic stress and immune response become mutually maintaining conditions, increasing the risk of inflammatory, neurodegenerative, and autoimmune diseases. Postpartum mothers experience stress, but lactation may act as a buffer between the stressor and the stress response.

Chapter 3. Introduction to Psychoneuroimmunology and the Immunology of Pregnancy and the Postpartum

In this chapter, we describe the scientific and theoretical framework for much of our thinking about maternal mood, stress, and lactation using research from psychoneuroimmunology (PNI). PNI describes a way of thinking about health that is very holistic and integrative. It attempts to understand and explain interactions between the biological substrate of brain and nervous system, endocrinology, and immunology and the "softer" elements–psychology, sociology, and spirituality. Based on discoveries made in the 70s and 80s about the anatomical links between the immune system and the nervous system, PNI views these interacting systems as an interconnected web or network. A small change or perturbation in one system could have multiple and far reaching effects on other systems. A change in an emotion, for example, would result in changes in neurological pathways, endocrine response, and, ultimately, immunity. PNI also tries to make sense of the well-known stress-illness relationship. Factors, such as personality, temperament, development, environment, and genetics, are all incredibly important to the biology of PNI.

Lactation is certainly a physiological phenomenon, but it is associated with multiple psychological and sociological demands, significances, and interactions. The importance of the health of the pregnancy in successful subsequent lactation and breastfeeding must be emphasized. For example, a woman may desire to breastfeed, be healthy, and may try to be successful. However, if she has had a stressful, unsupported pregnancy or illness during pregnancy, current little social support, or even a negative and disapproving family, the ability to even produce milk is threatened because of the well-known inhibitory effects of stress on the let-down reflex and the lesser well-known effects of stress on milk production and milk competency in general.

The stress women may feel under these circumstances could even translate into self-esteem problems, physical effects on health, and potential immune compromise. These effects then could ultimately affect the infant's health and well-being. In order for women to have a successful breastfeeding experience, nature has done its best to provide women with neuroendocrine and neuroimmune protections that promote lactation. These will be further described in chapters 3 and 5.

Interestingly, there has been little research on the psychoneuroimmunology of the postpartum in general, and lactation in particular. Yet it makes sense that nature would provide immunological protection for postpartum mothers, considering the survival of the species absolutely requires that newborns be protected from pathogens. The mother is the buffer between a potentially dangerous and threatening environment and the immunologically immature neonate. So, while nature has provided multiple mechanisms for protection of the infant (maternal antibodies crossing the placenta during pregnancy, the enteromammeric and bronchomammeric links), contact with a healthy and immunocompetent mother remains necessary for optimal protection of the newborn.

Yet mothers have gone through a period of immunocompromise during pregnancy, and have then experienced two recent enormously physically and emotionally stressful events: labor and birth. PNI would predict that the immune system of such a person could be threatened by these stressor effects. However, it seems that just the opposite is true for mothers across all societal ranges and privileges. Postpartum women seem especially protected from the ravages of stress! And lactating mothers' breastmilk seems to be immunologically preserved in even the worst circumstances. To understand and appreciate this remarkable phenomenon, we will review the basic tenets and findings of the field of PNI.

The History of Psychoneuroimmunology

There has truly been a revolution in the way scientists view the mind-body relationship. In the not very distant past, the possibility of a two-way interaction between the mind and the body was viewed skeptically. A dualistic perspective of health was the foundation of modern medicine, stemming from medieval concepts and the philosophy of René Descartes. There developed medical specialization upon specialization, with the body being divided up into systems, and then even further into parts of systems, with only one of the systems–psychiatry–devoted to the mind. This way of thinking was reinforced by the fact that many common diseases that physicians treated were caused by single entities: microbes. People died of infectious illnesses (pneumonia, influenza, tuberculosis, gastroenteritis) at the turn of the twentieth century. These were diseases that ultimately could be treated by "magic bullets" once antibiotics became widely available after WWII.

It is only in the last 50 years or so that the causes of most morbidity and mortality in the developed world have changed from infections to so-called lifestyle and chronic diseases: illnesses that are multifactorial and to a great extent self-inflicted by overnutrition, sedentariness, and dangerous health habits. These chronic diseases, such as cardiovascular diseases, obesity, type-2 diabetes, metabolic syndrome, and even cancer have both physical and genetic origins and behavioral and psychosocial roots. Medicine can no longer ignore the mind when, in fact, the mind is, in large part, directing one's health destiny. And clearly no magic bullet will be found to "cure" these illnesses.

Developing a holistic perspective of human health has not been a prerogative of healthcare specialties, as biological knowledge increased and biological variables became increasing analyzed into complex networks that were difficult to examine as whole systems. It was impossible for the average healthcare provider to "keep up" with the knowledge explosion. This fostered continuing compartmentalization of human health and healthcare.

Psychosomatic Symptoms

Yet, there was also a general acknowledgment that if a person presenting with a symptom could not be diagnosed by the modern tools available, the symptom potentially could be "all in your head." What that often meant was a conveyance of the belief that oftentimes the person was "faking" the symptom. This was a demeaning and frustrating perspective for such people who were truly suffering. Medicine just did not have the knowledge of neurochemistry, neurobiology, or psychoneuroimmunology to appreciate that the symptoms people reported were absolutely real, physical, and debilitating in many cases. These symptoms ultimately became known as psychosomatic: physical symptoms that somehow originated in the brain.

Conflicting evidence between the dualistic notions of modern medicine and the realities of people's health and illness experiences arose more and more frequently in the 1950s and 60s. Recognition of the role of stress in illness etiology or aggravation was becoming apparent. Certain diseases became known as stress-related, based in part on Hans Selye's description of the General Adaptation Syndrome (Selye, 1956). Certain "personalities" became known as disease-prone, such as the Type-A personality pattern and cardiovascular disease (Rosenman & Friedman, 1974), and the "rheumatoid arthritis" personality (Moos & Solomon, 1964).

Yet, even as recently as 1989, physicians did not appear to evaluate or acknowledge the significance of patients' stress experiences or levels when diagnosing them. Kroenke and Mangelsdorff (1989) did a retrospective chart review of 100 patients over three years seen at the Brooks Army Medical Clinic in San Antonio, Texas. Using a checklist of 14 common symptoms, they determined that 24% of the patients developed one symptom during the three year study period, 9% developed two symptoms, 3% developed three, and 2% developed four or more symptoms from the checklist. The patients were active duty, family members, and retired personnel. What makes their study so remarkable is that nearly three-fourths of the patients' symptoms could not be attributed to any organic disease etiology. These symptoms included chest pain, fatigue, dizziness, headache, leg swelling (edema), back pain, shortness of breath, insomnia, abdominal pain, numbness, erectile dysfunction, weight loss, cough, and constipation. So what caused these multiple, disparate symptoms? A second look at the lives of these individuals might reveal that stress could have played a significant role in symptomatology. But how does stress actually cause a physical symptom?

Stress and Immunity

Stressors are the triggers that elicit psychophysiological responses. And it is well known that individual's perceptions and appraisals of these stressors vary greatly, depending upon multiple factors. Life experiences, age, general health, genetics, reactivity, cognitive processes, behavioral patterns, and cultural and societal norms are just some of the factors that might influence how a person might respond to a particular stressor. These have been discussed in chapter 2. But for the stress/immune/disease links, what is important to understand is that an individual will launch a physiological stress response when the brain has processed information about the stressor and determined that there is threat or danger that needs a response. Once that stressor is translated into activation of the sympathetic adrenal medullary (SAM) system or the hypothalamic-hypophyseal-adrenocortical (HPA) systems, the potential for health effects through immune mechanisms exists. The SAM is designed to be a short-term alarm and arousal mechanism, but it can produce immune effects. HPA activation, a longer-term response, also has immune effects.

Stress that is ongoing, unremitting, and inescapable probably is the most damaging in terms of the immune system. This is particularly true if a person's coping mechanisms are inadequate to buffer the stress or if a person turns to unhealthy coping mechanisms that can actually aggravate and enhance the deleterious stress effects. The stress response itself can be damaging if not appropriately controlled. For example, an acute stress may translate into an inflammatory state that is activated to protect the individual. Chronic stress, on the other hand, may result in suppression of the adaptive, or specific, immune response. In order to understand these relationships, we will now describe the two arms of the immune system.

Inflammation and Innate Immunity

Overview of the Inflammatory Response

Inflammation is the body's ancient, rapid, and non-specific approach to threat, usually provoked by microbes, but also activated by sympathetic nervous system activation, and through other pathways. It is usually evoked in order to bridge the gap between the innate and specific immune responses and to destroy microorganisms through phagocytosis, activation of acute phase proteins, complement, chemotaxis, and vascular changes. If inflammation is not completely effective, the specific arm of the immune system acts to finish the work begun by inflammatory processes. Inflammation, therefore, is meant to be a short-term defense, basically acting to wall off infectious microbes and damaged tissue, remove these offenders from circulation and thus continual threat, and destroy them and repair the involved tissues.

The importance of this process is the recognition that human beings (and other animals) not only exist in a veritable sea of microorganisms, but contain within the body more microbial cells (10^{15}) than human cells (10^{14}) (Baron et al., 1996). Yet this is all usually balanced and safe because the innate response is incredibly vigilant and in almost all cases produces its protection without significant distinguishable biological signals. We are almost always totally unaware of the second-by-second battles launched by the innate immune system. In fact, when inflammation is clinically obvious, the battle has become a raging war.

Inflammatory mediators are powerful and non-specific, capable of destroying not only infected tissues, but potentially any cell populations. Inflammation is an imperfect system in that the natural controls and "stop-gaps" can be ineffective or overcome. A major cell type initiating inflammation is the macrophage. The products of activated macrophages are interleukin-1 (IL-1), interleukin-6 (IL-6), and tumor necrosis factor-α (TNF-α). One action of these proinflammatory cytokines is activation of the hypothalamic-hypophyseal-adrenocortical axis (HPA), a major stress pathway. The end product of this pathway is release of cortisol, which is a profoundly anti-inflammatory molecule. Thus, the inflammatory response is designed to be short lived, being down-regulated by cortisol, as well as by anti-inflammatory cytokines, such interleukin-10 (IL-10), transforming growth factor-ß (TGF-ß), a type of T cell known as the T-regulatory cell, and by the parasympathetic nervous system. This happens before tissue damage is excessive and by the time the specific immune response is responsive enough to launch its very directed attack against foreign or abnormal proteins.

Toll-Like Receptors

Macrophages, dendritic cells, granulocytes, and B lymphocytes have Toll-like receptors (TLRs), which respond to motifs of toxic microbial proteins, such as endotoxin, known as pathogen-associated microbial proteins (PAMPs). There have been 13 highly conserved TLRs identified, and they are found throughout the plant and animal kingdoms, and even on primitive invertebrates, such as insects. These TLRs have been conserved through evolutionary history and are obviously a critical component of an organism's defense. In lower animals, the innate response, initiated by binding of TLRs to PAMPs, is the only immune response possessed and is reasonably effective–but not perfect–in protecting the organism. These lower organisms sacrifice specificity of immune defenses, in part, because they produce huge numbers of progeny, which are part of food chains, and the majority of which, therefore, never develop into adult organisms. Contrast this to the comparatively small litters of mammals, or even the singleton births of humans. These progeny are precious to survival of the species and relying on innate, non-specific defense is not adequate. These higher organisms need a more effective system, and the specific immune response answers that need. The specific immune defense arose much later in evolution, but the innate response remains part of the human defense repertoire as the initial protection against microbes.

Innate immunity has become the focus of immunological research in the past 15 years because of the enormous body of evidence linking inflammation to many common human diseases. The various processes in the inflammatory response, if inappropriate, uncontrolled, excessive, or long-lasting, are the pathophysiological underpinnings of a long list of human illnesses.

The Innate Immune Response

Macrophages are ubiquitous phagocytic cells within tissues throughout the body. They arise from monocytes in the blood, which migrate through the endothelium into the interstitial spaces of all the tissues of the body. Signals initiating the macrophage-mediated innate immune response are illustrated in Figure 3-1, with the classical PAMPs-TLRs pathway highlighted. However, there are multiple pathways to activation. Macrophages have ß2 and α receptors on their cell surfaces which respond to epinephrine liberated from the adrenal gland by the sympathetic nervous system, another stress pathway. Heat shock proteins (HSPs) are released from damaged or traumatized cells, which are then capable of activation of the innate response. This type of tissue damage may not involve any type of microbial PAMPS. Other pathways include complement activation.

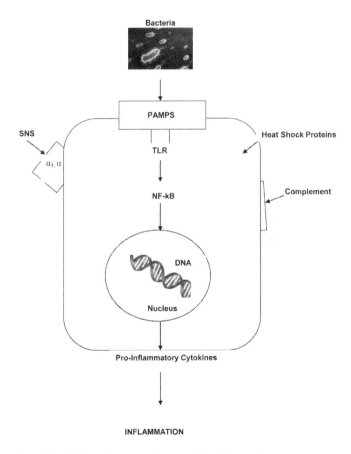

Figure 3-1. Signals initiating the macrophage-mediated innate immune response.

Pro Inflammatory Cytokines

Once activated, macrophages release a group of proinflammatory cytokines, once known as endogenous pyrogen (EP), consisting of IL-1, IL-6, and TNF-α. These cytokines are synthesized in cells through the activation of NF-kB, a transcription factor. The effects of these proinflammatory cytokines are autocrine, paracrine, and endocrine. A major effect is the pyogenic effect on the hypothalamus, acting through prostaglandin E2, causing resetting of the body's set point for body temperature, and thus inducing fever. Fever has been demonstrated to augment the body's immune response, by activating monocytes and enhancing neutrophil function (Rosenspire, Kindzelskii, & Petty, 2002). Yet fever can be maladaptive if too high, such as in sepsis. There appear to be natural molecules (cryogens) which balance the effects of pyrogens and regulate the degree of fever. These include α-MSH, arginine vasopressin, glucocorticoids, TNF, IL-10, and cytochrome P-450 (P-450), a component of the alternative pathway for arachidonic acid metabolism (Kozak et al., 2000).

The proinflammatory cytokines also act on other parts of the brain to induce a set of behaviors now considered protective, termed "sickness behavior." The characteristics of this syndrome are fatigue, excessive sleep, weakness, anorexia, lack of interest in social and sexual activities, muscle pain, and inability to concentrate. All of these behaviors are neurologically mediated and function to keep the infected individual metabolically and cognitively at rest, so presumably energy can be directed towards healing.

Acute-Phase Proteins

An additional response of the body to innate immune activation is release of acute-phase reactants. These molecules are primarily liberated from the liver in response to IL-6. These proteins rise in the plasma during acute inflammation to levels at least 25% greater than baseline, and include C-reactive protein (CRP) and coagulation factors, such as fibrinogen, amyloid, and complement components. The roles of these proteins are to opsonize bacteria (coat and thus label bacteria for later immune destruction) and to maintain the inflammatory state.

The Adaptive (Specific) Immune System

The goals of the innate response are to eliminate microbial invaders, but if not completely effective, the system also alerts and prepares the specific (adaptive) immune system. This system requires antigen presenting by various cells, such as macrophages, B cells, and most importantly, dendritic cells, which are widespread through the tissues and which are capable of traveling to lymph nodes, the sites of antigen presenting to T cells. These cells take up the antigen, break it into pieces, and then present the antigenic peptides in association with major histocompatibility complex (MHC) class II molecules on the cell surface to T helper lymphocytes, which have the appropriate T cell receptors (TCRs) for the particular peptides. This then is the signal for specific immune responses to follow, such as cell mediated cytotoxicity and B cell production of antibodies (Igs).

The innate immune response sets the stage for the adaptive immune system. Macrophages are involved in both responses. Complement, activated by the acute-phase protein CRP, when bound to antigenic material, can activate B lymphocytes. IL-6 inhibits T regulatory cells, so that the activation of the effector T cells is promoted. There is substantial cross-talk between these two branches of immunity in humans.

Chronic Stress and Inflammation

It can be seen from the above descriptions that the innate response is designed to be short term, and there is pathophysiological potential if the inflammatory mediators and processes are not appropriately halted. This appears to be the major problem in the many illnesses that appear to have a chronic inflammatory component. Other illnesses are characterized by recurring acute inflammatory signals. The presence of inflammation is often determined clinically by measuring cells (leukocytes) and sensitive acute-phase proteins and cytokines, with high-sensitivity (hs) CRP being the most common marker. Levels greater than 3 mg/L are considered to contribute to the prediction of CVD in patients with elevated low density lipoproteins (LDLs; Grundy et al., 2004). CRP is useful as a general, although non-specific marker of inflammation anywhere in the body. CRP is known to activate complement and causes expression of endothelial adhesion molecules (Pasceri, Willerson, & Yeh, 2000) and chemoattractants (Pasceri, Cheng, Willerson, & Yeh, 2001), and increases LDL uptake by macrophages (Zwaka, Hombach, & Torzewski, 2001).

Acute, and sometimes chronic, stress appears to be a potent inflammatory signal. In a sense, the body is readying itself to respond if a person is threatened and could potentially be injured in a stressful situation. Bleeding and infection would be inhibited by an acute inflammatory response. Of course, for humans, stressors nowadays are usually not dangers that would ultimately cause wounding and injury, but the stress response evolved over eons as a protective response to common dangers, such as predation. Today's stressors are as likely to be psychosocial as they are physical. But the body's response is fairly uniform once the brain has processed information and made a decision that a stress response is required. For humans, this stress response can even be elicited by mind alone. Imagination, perseveration, even dreaming can all lead to a perception of stress in the brain, translated into a neuroendocrine reaction, and even then into an inflammatory cascade of events.

The critical factor in whether stress can produce long-term pathophysiological change seems to be in the relationship between the inflammatory cascade and the natural opposing forces that are inhibitory brakes on inflammation. Thus, in a normal stress response activation of the HPA, the release of cortisol acts to suppress the inflammation. While we might expect to see chronic inflammation in diseases, such as rheumatoid arthritis, we also observe it in severe and chronic stress states, such as long-term depression or posttraumatic stress disorder. Why the HPA activation and release of cortisol is inadequate to suppress inflammation in these chronic stress states is perhaps related to glucocorticoid receptor (GR) sensitivity. If the GRs are downregulated and refractory to high levels of cortisol, then the inflammation can persist. Without a regulatory control on inflammation, there can be very significant cell damage to normal tissues. This could lead to inflammation that persists and damages tissues, such as endothelium, which could contribute to the development of atherosclerotic plaque.

Gender Differences in Immunity

There are significant gender differences in immunity and in the stress-immune relationship. The female hormone estrogen stimulates immune responses, while testosterone is immunosuppressive (Burger & Dayer, 2002). Thus, premenopausal females have more activated cellular and humoral immune responses than males. Females are more able to quickly heal wounds, produce immunoglobulins, and reject foreign tissue. Unfortunately, a side effect of this immune upregulation is a markedly higher risk for autoimmune diseases in females compared to males.

Pregnancy and Immunity

Another unique aspect of female life is the many changes that occur during different phases of childbearing. During pregnancy, there are enormous changes in immunity, which act to protect the developing semiallogeneic fetus from maternal immune recognition and destruction. The changes associated with pregnancy include decreased cellular (Th1) immunity and increased humoral (Th2) immunity, decreased Natural killer (NK) cell cytotoxicity, and enhanced innate (inflammatory) immune processes.

Pregnancy is truly unique from both immunological and PNI perspectives. The immune system in pregnancy is modified in many ways in order to prevent rejection of the semi-allogeneic fetus. Alterations in both adaptive and innate immune mechanisms vary throughout pregnancy, depending on trimester, exposures to microorganisms, preexisting conditions, and disease processes, such as preeclampsia or pregnancy-induced hypertension that might occur during the pregnancy (Mor & Cardenas, 2010).

Stress, anxiety, and depression also are factors than can alter the normal immune changes of pregnancy. Exactly how pregnancy affects the human immune system is still a mystery, but animal models are useful in examining how immunity does change. Murine models support the presence of a strong Th2 immune bias, but that has been less well documented in human pregnancies. In general, Th1 responses provoke cellular immunity and inflammatory reactions, and Th2 responses provoke humoral immunity and anti-inflammatory reactions (Raghupathy & Kalinka, 2008). In human pregnancies, the Th1 suppression and Th2 upregulation is thought to occur, but may change over the course of the pregnancy and may be regulated by familial and environmental factors (Halonen et al., 2009).

There is evidence that prenatal stress, anxiety, or depression influences the outcome of human pregnancies. For example, in a prospective study of 681 pregnant women from France, women who were depressed had more than triple the rate of preterm birth compared to non-depressed women (Dayan et al., 2006). All of the women enrolled in the study were considered low risk for preterm birth and were enrolled at 20 to 28 weeks gestation. Similarly, a study of 1,820 women in Baltimore found that those who had high levels of pregnancy-related anxiety had higher rates of preterm birth than those with low pregnancy-related anxiety (Orr, Reiter, Blazer, & James, 2007). These findings remained even after controlling for other risk factors for preterm birth. A study in the Netherlands of 8,052 women found that babies born to women with high depressive symptoms had increased risk of being small for gestational age (SGA) or having a low Apgar score (Goedhart et al., 2010). And a population study for 1,501,894 singletons born in Denmark from 1979 to 2004 found that maternal bereavement (particularly loss of a child) during pregnancy, or one year before pregnancy, was related to increased incidence of cerebral palsy in the children from the index pregnancy (Li et al., 2009).

One hypothesis of why inflammation would be related to these negative birth outcomes has to do with the role of cytokines in the maintenance of pregnancy (Coussons-Read, Okun, Schmitt, & Giese, 2005). Proinflammatory cytokines are chiefly known for their role in protecting against infection and healing wounds. However, IL-6, IL-8, and TNF-α are also involved in ripening the cervix. If the in utero environment is high in these levels due to prenatal depression, stress, or anxiety, the mother's body may be mistakenly signaling that it is time to have the baby— even if it is too early. In their study of 24 pregnant women, Coussons-Read et al. found that high prenatal stress was associated with high IL-6 and TNF-α levels.

Stage of pregnancy may also be a factor in cytokine ratios (Mor & Cardenas, 2010). These authors suggest that implantation, placentation, and first and early second trimester represent an "open wound," with activation of inflammatory processes. In mid-pregnancy, there is downregulation of these innate mechanisms, followed by upregulation when birth is imminent. The inflammation of pregnancy is a "sterile" inflammatory state (Challis et al., 2009). Generally accepted in recent years is the idea that an inflammatory state is actually necessary for a successful pregnancy and out-of-control inflammation may lead to pathophysiological events (Rusterholz, Hahn, & Holzgreve, 2007).

Inflammation in pregnancy may be sustained by alarm and danger signals through toll-like receptors (Challis et al., 2009). Further evidence for inflammatory upregulation comes from increased IL-6 and C-reactive protein plasma concentrations in pregnancy (Derzsy, Prohaszka, Rigo, Fust, & Molvarec, 2010), as well as many other acute-phase proteins (Haram, Augensen, & Elsayed, 1983). Regulation of this inflammatory state is essential, though, because excessive inflammation may lead to miscarriage. T-regulatory cells and inhibitory cytokines probably suppress excessive inflammation, as does the HPA during pregnancy. The placenta produces large amounts of corticotrophin-releasing hormone (CRH), so pregnant women have high blood levels of cortisol. Cortisol is a major regulator of the inflammatory state and may play a role in keeping pregnancy-associated inflammation in check (Mastorakos & Ilias, 2003). Of note for the future lactation success of women, cortisol elevation has been noted in prenatal depression (Field & Diego, 2008) and may potentially alter the normal state of inflammation. The roles of the immune and inflammatory changes in preparing the breasts during pregnancy for later lactation are unknown.

The Postpartum and Immunity

At birth, there is evidence of a natural and profound inflammatory response. Delivery is associated with increased serum levels of inflammatory cytokines, such as interleukin-6 (IL-6) and interleukin-1 (IL-1). A broad state of immune activation continues into the very early postpartum, as measured by levels of neopterin, soluble interleukin-2 (IL-2) receptor, and soluble CD8 antigen. The average CRP levels of 55 postpartum women at one week after delivery was 20.5 mg/L. IL-6 at one week postpartum was 7.2 pg/mL (Groer, 2011, unpublished data). These are both much higher than normal control group's levels. This inflammatory state may help the woman recover from the biological stress and injuries associated with birth, but little is known about the magnitude and length of such a state.

Groer's group completed a study of postpartum women measured cross-sectionally at four to six weeks after the birth (Groer et al., 2005). The study compared immune and inflammatory activation markers (serum cytokines IFN- γ, TNF-α, IL-6, IL-2, IL-10), neopterin, C-reactive protein (CRP), Epstein Barr viral capsid antigen Ig titer, and lymphocyte subset percentages in 181 postpartum women and compared these data to 33 control women. Postpartum women at this point in time had higher serum levels of IL-10 (p<.001), IFNγ (p<.001), IL-6 (p<.001), TNF-α(p<.001), neopterin (p<.001), and CRP (p<.001). The serum Th1/Th2 (IFN-γ/IL-10) ratio was higher for the postpartum group (p<.01). The lymphocyte proliferation with PHA was higher, and there were significant differences in lymphocyte subsets, with NK cells (p<.001) and CD8 cells (p<.001) significantly lower in postpartum women. Postpartum women reported far fewer and less severe symptoms of infectious illness compared to controls (p<.001).

These differences suggest that postpartum women have a more activated immune system and upregulated innate inflammatory response. The differences in lymphocytes population between postpartum and controls suggest the possibility of trafficking through increased extravasation of these cytotoxic cells into tissues, such as the involuting uterus. The higher levels of acute-phase reactants and proinflammatory cytokines suggest the possibility that there may be upregulated endothelial adhesion molecules in postpartum women. That evolution has endowed postpartum women with a vigorous inflammatory response is not surprising, considering that protection of the infant through nurturance and transfer of immune factors is almost entirely maternal in most species. What is surprising is that the length of the postpartum as a physiological state is not well defined, but most certainly lasts longer than the six weeks most American mothers take as maternity leave. After completing the initial study, we sought to analyze the longitudinal changes in postpartum women over the first postpartum year. We have now evidence that the postpartum is at least one year in length.

Groer's lab at the University of South Florida, College of Nursing in Tampa, Florida, is completing a NIH funded four year study of postpartum stress and immunity. We have followed 70 healthy women, starting at 16-25 weeks of pregnancy, and then at one week, and thereafter every month until the sixth postpartum month. Mothers complete a battery of stress and mood questionnaires, and blood is drawn for immune and endocrine analysis at every visit. We are very interested in the relationship of lactational state to stress in these mothers and will discuss these studies in Chapter 5.

Overall, our research has provided us with a longitudinal picture of how the immune system is changing over the postpartum, "recovering" from pregnancy. For example, the CRP levels, so extremely high right after birth, decline to normal slowly through the first postpartum year. Plasma levels of IL-6 are more variable than CRP, as it is a responsive cytokine to stress, circadian rhythms, and illnesses. Nevertheless, the mean level at birth was 7.2 pg/mL, and at six months postpartum, it was 4.3 pg/mL, a statistically significant drop over time.

Interestingly, the plasma IL-6 levels across the entire postpartum differ by breastfeeding status. There is a trend across the entire postpartum for breastfeeding women to have lower levels of this proinflammatory cytokine. The postpartum, therefore, seems to be characterized by an upregulated innate immune system, but formula-feeding women are in a higher inflammatory state. This may be due to a number of factors. Formula-feeding mothers tend to have higher stress and lower socioeconomic status in our sample. These factors will need to be controlled for as we complete data collection and analyses.

The adaptive immune system also is of interest. IFN-γ is a signature Th1 cytokine, which remains very low in plasma during pregnancy. Breastfeeding women appear to have lower IFN-γ levels during the early postpartum, suggesting that the Th1 axis, which is suppressed in pregnancy, continues to be suppressed for several months in breastfeeding women, and not in formula-feeding mothers. This is further supported by a shift towards IL-10, a regulatory and Th2 cytokine, that is much higher throughout the first five postpartum months in breastfeeding women. IL-10 may be active in suppressing the Th1 axis and decreasing inflammation. It may also be involved in regulating many aspects of the immune system, including cytotoxic cells.

One very surprising finding in our research has been the observation that Natural Killer cell (NKs) are markedly suppressed in the postpartum. Our earlier study found that NK cells percentages were lower in postpartum women than control women. In the current study, we are measuring exactly how cytotoxic these cells are in a culture designed to measure the ability of these cells to lyse a tumor cell line. Figure 3-2 depicts the NK cytotoxicity in lytic units across the postpartum. The control levels were measured in age matched non-pregnant, non-postpartum females compared to postpartum women. Across the postpartum, there is a suppression of NK cytotoxicity in postpartum women (Groer, El-Badri, Djeu, Harrington, & Van Eepoel, 2009)

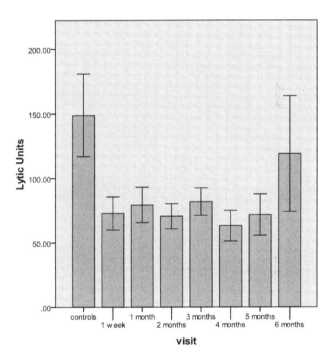

Figure 3-2. Lytic Units per 107 PBMCs in controls and postpartum women. Lytic Units were calculated from co-cultures of PBMCs, preincubated with rIL-2 for 18 hours, with Cr51-labeled K562 cells at 4 effector: target ratios. The cells were cultured together in RPMI for four hours, and the radioactivity in supernatants was counted and used in the calculation of lytic units. From Groer et al., 2009. Used with permission.

Our research suggests that the NK cell's inhibitory receptors are upregulated in postpartum women. Normal control plasma, when incubated with these cells, appears to further suppress cytotoxicity, but has no effect on control women's NK cytotoxicity. The NK cytotoxic function appears restored to control levels starting at six months postpartum.

It is curious that NK cytotoxicity is suppressed during a time when other protective mechanisms are enhanced, presumably to protect the mother and baby. NK cells act to lyse foreign cells, cancer cells, and virally infected cells. We have suggested that this suppression of NK cytotoxicity is similar to what is well known to occur in pregnancy: suppression so that NK cells do not attack fetal cells. Fetal cells travel through the placenta into the mother's circulation during pregnancy. These cells are stem cells of hematopoietic and mesenchymal origin and are known as fetal microchimeric cells (Groer, Manion, Szekeres, & El-Badri, 2011). They are recognized by the maternal immune system, but not attacked. It is now well established that these cells survive, and even thrive, for years in a mother's body, perhaps for her lifetime. Previously regarded as potentially dangerous propagators of autoimmune and even malignant disease, fetal microchimeric cells are now increasingly being recognized and analyzed for their healing, reparative, and even regenerative roles. So perhaps the establishment of tissue niches for these cells requires a continuation of the pregnancy-related NK cytotoxicity suppression until these cells have become well established. Lactational status does not seem to be a major factor in levels of NK cytotoxicity across the postpartum. However, breastmilk does contain maternal stem cells, and perhaps another source of microchimerism is through human milk.

Chapter 4. Lactational Stress Resistance

While mothers often experience many stressors in the postpartum period, nature has designed a way to potentially decrease the magnitude and distraction of the physiological stress response. Lactation is characterized by a unique endocrine and immune state, directed towards protection of the maternal-infant dyad from environmental stimuli and infectious agents. The neuroendocrine and neuroimmune changes at birth and during lactation may be adaptive, reducing maternal reactivity to the environment, promoting calmness and nurturing behavior, maintaining quantity and quality of milk, enhancing immune function, and opposing glucocorticoid mediated catabolism (Altemus, Deuster, Galliven, Carter, & Gold, 1995). It seems redundant to point out that only humans, among all mammals, choose *not* to lactate. It is not an option for any other mothers throughout the animal kingdom. Thus, it is of concern to apply data from the animal world to humans and their behaviors since postpartum women may fully formula feed, may exclusively lactate, may start breastfeeding and then stop, and may only partially breastfeed. So all mammalian mothers (except humans) exclusively lactate, as evolution designed them to. When examining the research on lactation in lower mammals, this point must be considered.

There is quite a bit of evidence that most lactating mammals exhibit markedly decreased stress responses in both the sympathetic nervous system (SNS) and hypothalamic-pituitary-adrenocortical (HPA) reactivity. Stress responsiveness does return very quickly when lactation ceases (Windle et al., 1997), as do corticotrophin-releasing hormone (CRH) and blood levels of cortisol, ACTH, and prolactin (Fischer, Patchev, Hellbach, Hassan, & Almeida, 1995). This decrease in stress reactivity appears to arise in late pregnancy. There is a surge of cortisol during the last stage of pregnancy due in part to placental corticotrophin-releasing hormone (CRH). Placental CRH inhibits hypothalamic CRH and stimulates both ACTH and glucocorticoid secretion.

At the end of pregnancy, mothers' cortisol levels are very high and may actually approach levels seen in clinical depression, anorexia nervosa, or strenuously exercising athletes (Magiakou, Mastorakos, Webster, & Chrousos, 1997). Cortisol facilitates many physiological and behavioral adaptations of pregnancy, including catabolic mobilization of maternal energy sources to meet fetal needs and preparation of the breasts for later lactation (Atkinson & Waddell, 1995).

As pregnancy advances, there is evidence that the usual effect of CRH on stimulating ACTH from the pituitary gland is decreased. It was found that the CRH receptor binding in the hypothalamus was decreased in pregnant rats compared to virgins (Neumann et al., 1998). Primates have elevated CRH during pregnancy, the origin of which is largely the placenta, which rises throughout pregnancy, peaks at labor, and falls dramatically at one day postpartum with the loss of the placental CRH (Smith, Chan, Bowman, Harewood, & Phippard, 1993).

When a protein increases markedly in the body, the receptor that it binds with often becomes downregulated: there is less synthesis by the DNA of the cells of the receptor. Elevated placental CRH in pregnancy results in decreased numbers and responsiveness of CRH receptors in the brain, and thus decreased release of ACTH and cortisol. This must "reset" after birth when there is an abrupt and dramatic decrease in CRH circulating in the woman's body.

The early postpartum is characterized by the very common occurrence of postpartum dysphoria, which may be due to the adjustment of the HPA to the non-pregnant state. Magiakou et al. (1997) found that women who developed dysphoria or depression were more likely to have longer and more severe postpartum periods of blunted ACTH response to exogenous CRH administration. In another study, lower levels of evening cortisol in the early postpartum period were associated with postpartum depression (Harris et al., 1996).

Pregnant women have a blunted ACTH secretion following stressor exposure in pregnancy, but they also have a tonically elevated glucocorticoid secretion, due to the very high drive provided by placental CRH. In this case, the high levels of cortisol result in downregulated cortisol receptors in the brain and pituitary, which normally are very responsive to blood cortisol, which acts to negatively feedback on the production of CRH and ACTH. Plasma cortisol levels in animals are not thought to be elevated in the postpartum, but there is evidence of reduced stress reactivity. Biological changes include decreased transcription of the CRH gene and decreased release of CRH, ACTH, cortisol, oxytocin, prolactin, and catecholamines in response to stressors. Behaviorally, mothers are less aggressive and anxious, quieter, and show exploratory and nurturing behaviors directed towards the infant pups (Shanks, Kusnecov, Pezzone, Berkun, & Rabin, 1997).

Animal Studies

The mechanisms through which the HPA axis is blunted to stress during lactation may be through neuroendocrinologic mechanisms. Estrogen is an important factor in the secretion of ACTH. Estrogen-responsive elements have been recently identified on the promotor region of the CRH gene, with estrogen directly stimulating CRH production (Magiakou et al., 1997). Thus, the low levels of estrogen during lactation may reduce CRH release in the brain. In addition, oxytocin and prolactin, which are high during lactation, may inhibit the HPA axis. Cook infused oxytocin and prolactin into both lactating and non-lactating sheep exposed to a stressor (a barking dog). Cortisol release was decreased in both (Cook, 1997).

The central mechanisms by which HPA reactivity is blunted have been thought to include other mechanisms, such as the SNS. Windle et al. (1997) found that noradrenergic activation of the HPA axis was significantly reduced in lactating rats. Intracerebroventricular injection of the α1-sympathetic agonist methoxamine resulted in increased plasma cortisol in virgin rats, but not in lactating rats. Methoxamine also induced CRF messenger RNA expression in the brain of virgin rats, but not in lactating rats. The data suggest that there is a suppression of noradrenergic activation of the HPA axis in lactating animals. These results were confirmed by Toufexis and Walker (1996) who showed that stimulatory SNS innervation of the hypothalamic neurons that secrete CRH facilitated ACTH responses to stress in virgin rats, but not to lactating rats.

In another experiment, cfos mRNA expression was measured in brains of lactating compared to virgin female rats exposed to immobilization stress (da Costa, Wood, Ingram, & Lightman, 1996). cfos mRNA expression is a general measure of stress-induced neuronal activation and was diminished in the hypothalamic CRH secreting neurons (paraventricular nucleus or "PVN") of lactating rats. cfos mRNA expression was also reduced in the medial amygdala, lateral septum, and cingulate cortex, suggesting the attenuation of stress responsiveness in lactating animals was due to inhibition of afferent pathways to the PVN.

Plasma catecholamines also appear to be reduced in response to stressors in lactating rats. Immobilization stress produced a significantly smaller elevation in both plasma epinephrine and norepinephrine in lactating compared to non-lactating diestrous rats. Of note is that plasma prolactin increased in non-lactators, but did not change in lactating stressed rats (Higuchi, Negoro, & Arita, 1989). Lightman and Young (1989) showed a similar effect on oxytocin release in stressed lactating rats.

Windle et al. (1997) discovered a difference in behavioral responses to stressors in lactating rats. In response to ten minutes of white noise (a mild stressor), virgin rats showed HPA activation and increased activity levels, displacement grooming behaviors, and rearing, while lactating rats showed a different repertoire of behaviors that were directed towards the pups. These same rats did not show activation of the HPA axis in response to white noise, indicating a possible dissociation between the behavior and the neuroendocrine biology. During lactation there may also be increased levels of the major inhibitory neurotransmitter in the brain, gamma amino butyric acid, which may behaviorally inhibit the affective state of the lactating animal (Qureshi, Hansen, & Sodersten, 1987).

While the lactational stress resistance in rodents appears to dominate perinatal behavior, when the mother senses real threat to herself and her pups, she does respond appropriately (Deschamps, Woodside, & Walker, 2003). When exposed to a male predator or the scent of fox urine, mother rats launched a stress response and displayed aggressive behavior. Interestingly, the presence of the pups was absolutely required for the stress hyporesponsivity; if they were removed, the stress reactivity returned to levels of virgin rats.

In a recent report of stress and immunity in lactating and non-lactating female rats, lactating rats differed in that prior to stress exposure they had higher granulocyte counts and lower IL-2 production. A confrontational stress paradigm produced a drop in granulocytes and IL-2 in non-lactating rats, but this did not occur in the lactating rats (Jaedicke, Fuhrmann, & Stefanski, 2009).

Studies with Human Mothers

Very little research has been done on the reactivity to stressors in lactating humans. In a study reported in 1995, 20 minutes of graded treadmill exercise was used as a stressor in ten lactating vs. ten non-lactating women. The lactating women showed lower plasma levels of ACTH, cortisol, glucose, and norepinephrine (Altemus et al., 1995). In contrast, exhaustive treadmill exercise in 17 lactating women markedly decreased the milk concentration of Immunoglubulin A(IgA) during the 30 minutes post-exercise (Gregory, Wallace, Gfell, Marks, & King, 1997). These authors suggested that there is an accumulation of lactic acid in milk after exercise, which then degraded secretory Immunoglobulin (sIgA), but the role of adrenergic arousal and stress hormones on milk sIgA were not discussed.

Several studies of cardiovascular function during lactation have been done. In one study of mothers in the laboratory, systolic blood pressure (BP) was lower after baby contact. Breastfeeding mothers had lower BP during stress sessions and after baby feeding at home. Oxytocin was measured in this study and results suggested that oxytocin has anti-stress and blood pressure lowering effects (Light et al., 2000). Mezzacappa and colleagues (2001) found that breastfeeding women showed evidence of a shift towards parasympathetic nervous system dominance compared to bottle-feeding women. More frequent feeding was a critical factor in breastfeeding effects on autonomic nervous system balance.

Depressed and non-depressed mothers who were breastfeeding compared to bottle-feeding mothers were reported to show more relaxation and less burping and intrusive behaviors with their three-month-old infants (Field et al., 2010). Of interest is a report that breastfed compared to formula-fed infants had higher salivary cortisol (Cao et al., 2009), an anti-intuitive finding that was explained as the physical exertion of suckling in the breastfeeding infants, which produced a stress response. It was suggested that this stress response is actually of benefit for long-term health, in that it may impact development of the stress response and resilience later in life.

One study disputes the presence of a general hyporesponsivitivy of the HPA axis in lactating women (Meinlschmidt, Martin, Neumann, & Heinrichs, 2010). These investigators stressed mothers with the Trier social stress test. Both breastfeeding and holding the infant produced decreases in ACTH, plasma cortisol, and salivary cortisol. They concluded that the restraint of the HPA occurs only short term, during the actual time of suckling.

In another study involving non-human primates, cortisol was higher in lactating free-ranging rhesus macaques measured after capture with their pups. The presence of the pups seemed to drive the stress responsivity in this study (Maestripieri, Hoffman, Fulks, & Gerald, 2008).

The act of suckling produces decreases in both ACTH and cortisol, which is contributed to by skin-to-skin contact (Handlin et al., 2009), and increases in prolactin, oxytocin, and β-endorphin are reported to occur during the act of breastfeeding (Franceschini et al., 1989). Bridges and colleagues (Byrnes, Rigero, & Bridges, 2000) found that blocking opioid receptors resulted in longer bouts of nursing in lactating rats. It was suggested that the mother engaged in nutritive and non-nutritive sucking in response to expectation that suckling would produce a sense of satisfaction that was blocked by the drug.

Mezzacappa and Katkin (2002) presented data from two studies that indicated that breastfeeding buffers mothers against negative mood. In the first study, they compared 20 breastfeeding and 27 bottle-feeding mothers on levels of perceived stress in the past month. As predicted, the breastfeeding mothers reported less stress, even after controlling for possible confounding variables.

The second study included 28 mothers who were both breast- and bottle-feeding (Mezzacappa & Katkin, 2002). The researchers measured mothers' stress levels immediately before and after both types of feeding. This study was a major methodological improvement over previous studies in that women served as their own controls. Since there were not pre-existing differences between breast- and bottle-feeding mothers, it was possible to attribute the observed difference in mood to feeding method alone. The researchers found that breastfeeding decreased negative mood and bottle feeding decreased positive mood in the same women.

A study of 43 breastfeeding women found that both breastfeeding and holding their babies without breastfeeding significantly decreased ACTH, plasma cortisol, and salivary free cortisol (Heinrichs et al., 2001). Breastfeeding and holding the infant led to significantly decreased anxiety, whereas mood and calmness improved only in the breastfeeding group. In response to an induced stressor, breastfeeding exerted a short-term suppression of the HPA axis response to mental stress. The authors concluded that suckling provided a short-term suppression of the stress-related cortisol response and HPA axis response to mental stress. They argued that this short-term suppression provided several evolutionary and biological advantages. It isolated the mothers from distracting stimuli, facilitated their immune system, protected the babies from high cortisol in the milk, and prevented stress-related inhibition of lactation.

In a study of lab-induced stress, breastfeeding women had a significantly attenuated stress response (Altemus et al., 1995). There were ten breastfeeding and ten non-breastfeeding women who were all seven to 18 weeks postpartum. They performed a 20-minute treadmill exercise program at 90% of maximal oxygen capacity in order to measure stress. Plasma ACTH, cortisol, and glucose were significantly lower in the breastfeeding vs. non-breastfeeding mothers. The same was true of basal norepinephrine. But overall sympathomedullary responses were similar in both groups. Prolactin levels were elevated throughout the exercise condition for breastfeeding women, and there was a difference in prolactin levels over time between the groups. Oxytocin levels did not change.

A large epidemiological study's results were that bottle-feeding mothers had higher scores on the Edinburgh Postnatal Depression Scale than breastfeeding mothers in 2,375 postpartum women (Warner, Appleby, Whitton, & Faragher, 1996). Our research group found that depressive symptoms at around four weeks postpartum were associated with lower morning salivary cortisol levels in postpartum mothers, although breastfeeding mothers had less depressive symptoms than bottle-feeding women (Groer & Morgan, 2007). The relationship between the neuroendocrinology of lactation and the development of postpartum depression is not clearly elucidated. Parity may be a mediator between breastfeeding and reduced risk of postpartum depression, with breastfeeding multiparas appearing more protected than primiparas (Sibolboro Mezzacappa & Endicott, 2007). Depression will be discussed in more detail in Chapter 5.

The difference in the HPA axis in lactating mothers compared to non-lactating women may protect mothers from the abrupt withdrawal of cortisol at birth and a rapid change in responsiveness of the CRH neuron when placental CRH is withdrawn. The role of prolactin and oxytocin in this process may be critical since both hormones suppress ACTH release. These, of course, are much lower in formula-feeding mothers compared to breastfeeding mothers.

It is interesting to note that the drug bromocriptine was frequently administered to human mothers in the past to suppress lactation, through its action as an inhibitor of prolactin release from the pituitary. There are reports of psychiatric disturbances in women receiving bromocriptine postpartum (Morgans, 1995). Could this be due to abrupt pharmacological withdrawal of prolactin's inhibition of the HPA axis?

Stress Hormones and Lactation

Cortisol

Cortisol is the major glucocorticoid released through activation of the HPA axis in humans. There is a possible period of hypocortisolemia immediately after birth, which is then followed by normal levels and circadian rhythms in the postpartum mother (Elenkov, Hoffman, & Wilder, 1997). However, the lactating mother would be presumed to have less of a response to stress-induced HPA or adrenergic arousal compared to non-lactating women.

Prolactin

Prolactin is another essential hormone for successful breastfeeding, as it controls milk synthesis. The stimulus for its release by the anterior pituitary includes suckling, proximity of the infant(s), and skin-to-skin contact. While prolactin levels drop over the course of lactation, the basal level remains higher than in non-lactating mothers. Oxytocin stimulates prolactin synthesis in the pituitary gland, but it is not known if it acts as a releasing hormone for prolactin. Prolactin is a trophic hormone, stimulating cell division and growth in several targets (breast, monocytes, and lymphocytes). Both oxytocin and prolactin increase the repertoire of maternal behaviors in lactating animals (Bosch, 2011). Prolactin is considered to function as a stress hormone under certain circumstances, and to have significant immune effects, depending upon concentration, but there are important differences in lactating animals, as they have higher baseline levels of prolactin in the *non-stressed* state. Stress produces a serum prolactin increase in non-lactating rats, while lactators have a decreased prolactin release. Prolactin is also known to suppress ACTH and promote Th1 mediated immune responses. Prolactin receptors exist on lymphocytes. Prolactin is a trophic hormone, stimulating cell division and growth in several targets (breast, monocytes, and lymphocytes). "Optimal" amounts of prolactin appear to be necessary for immune function. Both prolactin and oxytocin are hormones with physiological and behavioral effects. Prolactin and oxytocin have been shown to increase the repertoire of maternal behaviors in lactating animals.

Oxytocin

A central hormone in the dyadic interaction between a breastfeeding mother and her infant is oxytocin. While well known for its role in milk ejection and uterine contractions, oxytocin has many additional critical roles in behavior, stress reactivity, cardiovascular and nervous system functioning, endocrine responses, and immune function. Oxytocin appears to be essential for the development of maternal behavior and for bonding between mother and infant (and may be the pivotal mediator for the decreased stress reactivity, stress perception, lower blood pressure, and increased vagal tone that have been found in lactating mothers (Light et al., 2000).

A potent and well-known stimulus for pulsatile oxytocin release is suckling. If a poor latch and inadequate, weak suckling are present, then oxytocin release is decreased, and milk ejection is insufficient. However, breastfeeding is a somatosensory experience that involves more than nipple stimulation. There is skin contact and sensations of texture, size, and warmth, conscious and unconscious perceptions, such as odors and tastes, and a plethora of emotional responses. Human mothers frequently kiss their babies as they interact with them, a behavior which perhaps is analogous to the licking that is required behavior by rat mothers in order to develop the full array of maternal behavior, including lactation.

All of these inputs are important for lactation success and probably play some role in oxytocin release. Oxytocin release in human mothers was increased over pre-partal levels by early skin-to-skin contact (first two hours after birth; Nissen, Lilja, Widstrom, & Uvnas-Moberg, 1995). Oxytocin was shown to be released by electrical stimulation of afferent nerve fibers originating in the skin (Stock & Uvnas-Moberg, 1988) and by massage (Agren, Lundeberg, Uvnas-Moberg, & Sato, 1995). Other stimuli reported to increase oxytocin levels include touch, warmth, vibration, and electroacupuncture (Uvnas-Moberg, 1997). In fact, a nursing mother merely has to think about nursing her infant to induce a pulse of oxytocin and a subsequent let-down of milk. Thus, oxytocin release during maternal-infant interaction involves a multitude of psychological and sensory stimuli and is not confined just to the nipple.

Oxytocin has many prosocial and anti-stress effects in animal models (both male and female). In a review of behavioral effects of lactational hormones, Carter and Altemus (1997) propose that oxytocin and vasopressin are antagonistic, and that oxytocin opposes the defense reactions associated with stress, functionally antagonizing vasopressin's effects. Oxytocin promotes nurturance and maternal behaviors, lactation, anabolism, and energy conservation, and participates in the stress downregulation of lactation. When a mother is severely threatened, however, vasopressin release would override oxytocin's effects, allowing for flight-or-flight defensive responses of the threatened organism. Interestingly, oxytocin and vasopressin differ chemically from each other in only two amino acids.

Oxytocin is a non-peptide hormone synthesized in the hypothalamus. Oxytocin produced by the magnocellular neurons is transported to the posterior pituitary and released in a burst-like pulsatile pattern in response to somatosensory stimulation. The parvocellular oxytocinergic neurons remain and terminate within the brain and spinal cord, so oxytocin is available to act centrally as a neurotransmitter, as well as being secreted into the bloodstream from the posterior pituitary to act systemically (Uvnas-Moberg, 1997).

Oxytocin and Decreased Stress Reactivity

It is believed that oxytocin is an important mediator in the decreased stress responsiveness of animal mothers, with a great majority of studies done on lactating rats. Oxytocin acts on receptors throughout the hippocampus, hypothalamus, and limbic system, with a general effect of promoting calmness, increasing affiliative and nurturing behavior, and producing social responsivity (Uvnas-Moberg, 1997). In lactating rats, oxytocin's effects may be both energy saving (sedation, decreased reactivity, increased digestion and anabolic metabolism, decreased blood pressure) and energy transferring (milk ejection, cutaneous vasodilation, and increased levels of glucose and glucagon). Estrogen and progesterone during the last part of pregnancy activate the release of oxytocin that then affects maternal behavior in the early postpartum period. In lab animals with high levels of infanticide, infusion of oxytocin suppresses this behavior markedly (McCarthy, 1990).

While oxytocin appears responsible for initiating steroid dependent maternal behavior, it is not required to maintain it. Blocking oxytocin's effects by infusion of an oxytocin receptor antagonist into the cerebral ventricles of virgin and lactating rats resulted in increased concentrations of ACTH and corticosterone only in lactating rats (Neumann, Torner, & Wigger, 2000). When the animals were stressed, only virgin rats treated with the oxytocin receptor antagonist had an increase in ACTH and corticosterone. In addition, an anxiolytic effect of oxytocin has been found (Slattery & Neumann, 2010).

Another mechanism of importance in oxytocin's effect on stress reactivity appears to be through vagal mechanisms. Parasympathetic dominance characterizes the basal autonomic tone of the breastfeeding mother, and this may be through central stimulation of vagal efferent pathways that are affected by oxytocin, as well as by other inputs (e.g., gut cholecystokinin). This activity contributes not only to diminished stress reactivity, but also to lower blood pressure, greater lymphocyte responses to mitogens, and decreased cardiac variability in the basal state. The cardiovascular effects of oxytocin include not only the aforementioned vagal effects, but also natriuresis and vascular relaxation probably mediated through atrial natriuretic factor (Gutkowska, Jankowski, Mukaddam-Daher, & McCann, 2000). These researchers have also shown that oxytocin is actually synthesized in the heart where it acts on oxytocin receptors to decrease heart rate and force of contraction. Breastfeeding mothers have been reported to have higher vagal tone, as estimated from respiratory sinus arrhythmia (Redwine, Altemus, Leong, & Carter, 2001). Massage on the ventral surface of rats produced a long-lasting drop in blood pressure and heart rate (Lund, Lundeberg, Kurosawa, & Uvnas-Moberg, 1999), possibly through vagal mechanisms.

Groer's research has examined the psychoneuroendocrinology pathways in lactating women, using measures of life stress and perceived stress, and comparing exclusively lactating to exclusively formula-feeding women at four to six weeks postpartum. Breastfeeding mothers had more positive moods, reported more positive events, had lower depression and anger, and perceived less stress than formula-feeding women. There were few correlations among stress, mood, and the hormones in postpartum mothers, and those only in formula-feeders. Postpartum mothers reported a range of stress and negative moods at four to six weeks, and in formula-feeding mothers, serum prolactin was related to some of the stress and mood variables. Breastfeeding appears to be somewhat protective of negative moods and stress. The highest and lowest deciles on stress and mood scores in all mothers were compared for cortisol, ACTH and prolactin. Cortisol and ACTH were not statistically significantly different when deciles were compared by traditional parametric statistics (t-tests). However, since the variances were not equal, a Bayesian analysis, using the Behrens-Fisher distribution, found that the odds of elevated cortisol in the highest depression decile were greater than 6:1. For prolactin, there were statistically significantly different levels between the highest and lowest deciles for depression (p=.03), anxiety (p=.01), anger (p=.000), and total mood disturbance (p=.003), with the highest deciles having the lowest levels of prolactin. In these cases, prolactin is at least partly a surrogate for breastfeeding (Groer, 2005).

Conclusion

There is clear evidence for a significant reduction in stress responsivity in lactating animals. This reduction is reactivity is likely to be protective for both mother and infant, as metabolic energy is carefully conserved for the functions of nurturance and lactation. Nevertheless, mothers are able to launch a stress response when significantly threatened. Human mothers also appear to have diminished stress reactivity, although the picture is not as clear as in the animal world. Research suggests that the presence of the infant or the actual act of breastfeeding may be an essential component of the decrease in stress responsiveness. In tandem with this is the fact that lactating mothers can become aggressive and defensive when their infants are threatened.

Chapter 5. Breastfeeding, Mental Health, and the Lifetime Risk of Cardiovascular Disease and Metabolic Syndrome

Negative emotions, such as depression, anxiety, pessimism, hopelessness, anger, and shame, have a well-documented deleterious effect on health (Frazure-Smith & Lesperance, 2005; Kubzansky, Davidson, & Rozanski, 2005; Surtes et al., 2008). Specifically, negative emotional states have been related to increased risk of heart disease, metabolic syndrome and diabetes, cancer, and neurodegenerative diseases, such as Alzheimer's and multiple sclerosis. The mechanism for this link appears to be that these emotional states upregulate the stress response, particularly the inflammatory response system. Danese and colleagues (2009) note that depression, inflammation, and metabolic risk markers indicate stress-sensitive systems are functioning abnormally, and these three markers are good predictors of disease.

In this chapter, we describe three common causes of premature mortality for women–heart disease, metabolic syndrome, and diabetes–and how breastfeeding protects women's health because it lowers the risk of negative mental states and downregulates the stress response.

Depression

Depression is one of the most common of all mood disorders, and it is the mental state with the most clearly documented impact on health (Frasure-Smith & Lesperance, 2005; Kiecolt-Glaser et al., 2005; Pace et al., 2007; Wilson, Finch, & Cohen, 2002). Depression is twice as prevalent in women as it is in men, but that it affects the health of both men and women has been well-established. For example, in a large study of U.S. veterans (N=35,715), depressed patients were at increased risk of dying over a five year period (Kinder et al., 2008). This was not true for patients with posttraumatic stress disorder (PTSD) only or for those who had neither depression nor PTSD. The most often studied aspect of this relationship is the impact of depression on the inflammatory response, which has direct relevance for understanding the link between depression and heart disease.

Depression has also been implicated in the etiology of metabolic syndrome and diabetes. Researchers have specifically examined the relationship between depression and lipid profiles, triglycerides, and obesity. Of particular interest is the relationship between depression and visceral obesity, the type most likely to have a negative impact on health.

Depression and Inflammation

When first described more than a decade ago, researchers noted that high levels of proinflammatory cytokines increased the risk of depression (Maes & Smith, 1998), and this increase can be caused by psychological stress (Kendall-Tackett, 2007a). As is true of inflammatory diseases, the proinflammatory cytokines identified most often in depression are interleukin-1ß (IL-1ß), interleukin-6 (IL-6), and tumor necrosis factor-α (TNF-α). Researchers sometimes include other measures of inflammation in their studies. These include interferon-γ (IFN-γ), intercellular adhesion molecule (ICAM), or C-reactive protein (CRP; Pace et al., 2007). Fibrinogen, a soluble protein that aids in clotting, is another marker of inflammation. Because it increases the speed of platelet aggregation and thrombus formation, a high level of fibrinogen is a risk factor for cardiovascular disease and predicts cardiac events. Maes (2001) described the stress-depression-inflammation connection as follows:

> The discovery that psychological stress can induce the production of proinflammatory cytokines has important implications for human psychopathology and, in particular, for the aetiology of major depression. Psychological stressors, such as negative life events, are emphasized in the aetiology of depression. Thus psychosocial and environmental stressors play a role as direct precipitants of major depression or they function as vulnerability factors which predispose humans to develop major depression. Major depression is accompanied by activation of the inflammatory response system (IRS) with, among other things, an increased production of proinflammatory cytokines, such as IL-1ß, IL-6, TNF-α and IFN-γ, signs of monocytic- and T-cell activation, and an acute-phase response (Maes, 2001, p. 193).

In a recent meta-analysis of 136 studies, Howren, Lamkin, and Suls (2009) noted that all three inflammatory markers they studied (C-reactive protein, IL-1, and IL-6) were positively associated with depression. They found that this relationship was found in both clinical and community samples, and concluded that there was a dose-response effect: the higher the depression, the higher the inflammation. They also noted that there was a bidirectional relationship between depression and inflammation, with depression increasing inflammation and inflammation increasing depression.

How Depression Influences Health

Depression is a robust risk factor for cardiovascular disease, cardiovascular events, and cardiac-related mortality (Frasure-Smith & Lesperance, 2005; Kendall-Tackett, 2007b; Kendall-Tackett, 2009; Rutledge et al., 2006). Depressed patients have more frequent and earlier hospital readmissions and are more likely to have a number of behavioral risk factors, including smoking, obesity, and a sedentary lifestyle (Rieckman et al., 2006). The risk was not only for those suffering from major depression, but for milder forms as well. Behavior alone cannot account for the increased risk. Depression changes the inflammatory response system, which influences cardiac risk.

Depression, Inflammation and Heart Disease

Inflammation is a crucial factor in atherogenesis and the progression of coronary artery disease (Zouridakis, Avanzas, Arroyo-Espliguero, Fredericks, & Kaski, 2004). Inflammatory factors are not simply markers. They have a pathogenic role to play. And these inflammatory markers, including C-reactive protein and proinflammatory cytokines, are often elevated in depressed people.

Several studies have found elevated C-reactive protein in depressed patients with heart disease. In a study of men and women at risk for heart disease (N=68), Taylor and colleagues (2006) found that depressed patients, with a mean age of 62, had elevated C-reactive protein compared to the controls. The depressed patients also had abnormally low cortisol levels in response to stress, and a lower respiratory sinus arrhythmia. Coaguability may also be a factor in depression's impact on heart disease. A study of patients 65 and older found that depression was related to both C-reactive protein and coagulation factors (Kop et al., 2002). This study included 4,268 patients who were free of cardiovascular disease (mean age=72.4 years). Depressed men and women had elevated C-reactive protein, elevated white blood cell count, and increased markers of coaguability.

Similarly, coagulation was also related to depression and cardiovascular risk in a study of 3,292 perimenopausal women (Matthews et al., 2007). This study included five markers of hemostasis and inflammation. Over the five year period, once adjusting the model for health history, medication use, ethnicity, and menopausal status, depressive symptoms were related to fibrinogen and PAI-1. C-reactive protein was not elevated in women with depressive symptoms. The authors concluded that depressive symptoms may be associated with increased cardiovascular risk through hypercoagulability.

Depression has also been related to cardiac-related mortality risk. It predicted cardiac symptoms in a sample of 750 middle-aged women with suspected myocardial ischemia (Rutledge et al., 2006). Both treatments for depression and current depression severity were related to cardiac symptoms and outcomes over the course of the 2.3 year follow-up. The more severe the depression, the higher the mortality risk; each point increase on the Beck Depression Inventory was associated with a three percent increase in mortality risk, even after adjusting for age, disease severity, and other coronary artery disease risk factors.

In a study of survival after acute myocardial infarction (MI), 370 patients with an initial episode of major depression were compared with 550 with recurrent depression and 408 patients who were free of depression (Carney et al., 2009). The researchers found that those who had either initial or recurrent depression had shorter survival time following an acute MI than those with no depression. Initial episodes were more predictive of mortality than recurrent episodes, and this difference could not be explained by other risk factors.

Eighteen patients with congestive heart failure and depressive symptoms were enrolled in the study, and levels of IFN-γ, IL-6, and IL-10 CD4+ T cells were assessed (Redwine et al., 2007). The researchers found that higher depressive symptoms led to a prospective increase in cardiac rehospitalization or death over a two year period. Lower IFN-γ and anti-inflammatory IL-10 were prospectively related to increased depressive symptoms, cardiac rehospitalization, or death. Contrary to expectation, they did not find that IL-6 was elevated in depressed patients.

Treating depression without addressing inflammation may not be sufficient to reverse cardiac risk. In a sample of 129 patients with heart failure, soluble TNF-α levels were significantly higher in depressed versus non-depressed patients, and also for a subgroup of patients who were no longer depressed, but were on antidepressant medications (Moorman et al., 2007). These findings suggest that medications were treating depression, but not adequately reversing inflammation. There were no significant differences between the depressed and non-depressed groups in IL-1ß or IL-6.

The relationship between cardiovascular risk and depression also appears to be bidirectional. In a recent study of 824 young adults in Finland, the participants were recruited at ages three to eight years and followed for 21 years. Elovainio and colleagues (2010) noted that when the trajectory of triglycerides increased steeply over the lifespan, the steep trajectory was associated with higher depressive symptoms in adulthood. This relationship continued to exist even after controlling for other risk factors. The link between triglycerides and depression accounted for the relationship between depression and high BMI. The authors hypothesized that this pattern may also be one link between obesity and depressive symptoms.

Depression, Metabolic Syndrome, and Diabetes

Depression is also related to increased risk of metabolic syndrome and diabetes. Metabolic syndrome is the precursor syndrome to type-2 diabetes. It includes a cluster of symptoms: insulin resistance, high LDL and VLDL cholesterol, high triglycerides, and visceral obesity (Haffner & Taegtmeyer, 2003). Inflammation is related to metabolic syndrome and insulin resistance, which is related to an increased risk of cardiovascular disease.

For example, Vaccarino and colleagues (2009) found that in women with suspected coronary artery disease, depression was associated with about 60% increased odds for metabolic syndrome, and depression more than doubled their risk for cardiovascular disease over the 5.9 year follow-up. The sample was 652 women who participated in the Women's Ischemia Syndrome Evaluation (WISE) study. Both metabolic syndrome and depression were independently related to increased risk.

Another study found that depressive symptoms were related to visceral fat in middle-aged women (Everson-Rose et al., 2009). The sample included 409 women (45% African American, 55% White) who comprised the Chicago cohort of the Study of Women's Health Across the Nation (SWAN) study. They noted that women with clinically relevant depressive symptomatology had 24.5% more visceral fat than women who were not depressed. There was no difference based on depressive symptomatology for subcutaneous fat, which is not considered a risk factor for cardiovascular disease. The authors concluded that visceral fat was another pathway by which depression contributes to increased risk of obesity and cardiovascular disease.

In a study of women in the Pittsburgh cohort of the SWAN study (35% African American), researchers found that for women free of metabolic syndrome at the outset of the study, either a lifetime history of major depression or current depression predicted metabolic syndrome at the follow-up (Goldbacher, Bromberger, & Matthews, 2009). A lifetime history of alcohol abuse or dependence also independently predicted metabolic syndrome, but attenuated the relationship between depression and metabolic syndrome. The authors noted that interventions that address depression may well prevent the onset of metabolic syndrome.

A study of 921 men and women from Finland also found a relationship between depression and metabolic syndrome, but for women only (Pulkki-Raback et al., 2009). Women with depressive symptoms had an increased risk of metabolic syndrome. Metabolic syndrome in childhood predicted higher depressive symptoms in adulthood. In a sample of 4,641 middle-aged women (mean age=52 years), researchers found that a history of childhood physical or sexual abuse doubled the risk of both depression and obesity (Rohde et al., 2008).

Depression in patients who already have type-2 diabetes increases mortality risk from a wide variety of causes. In a prospective study of 4,184 patients with type-2 diabetes, 581 died over the study period (Lin et al., 2009). A significantly higher number of patients with either major or minor depression (17.8% and 18.2%, respectively) died compared to 12.9% of patients with no depression. The causes of death included cardiovascular disease (43%), cancer (27%), or "other" (31%), which included infections, dementia, renal failure, and chronic obstructive pulmonary disease. The authors concluded that for patients with diabetes and comorbid depression, risk of mortality increased substantially from causes above and beyond cardiovascular disease.

Summary

Depression is associated with increased levels of C-reactive protein and other markers of inflammation, such as coaguability. Not surprisingly, it is related to heart disease and predicts new cardiac events. Depression also predicts metabolic syndrome and diabetes, and premature mortality. Unfortunately, depression is not alone in increasing risk of disease. Hostility is a related mental state that also increases risk for both cardiac and metabolic diseases.

Hostility

For those with a hostile world view, life is not benign. Hostile people don't trust others, are suspicious and cynical about human nature, and have a tendency to interpret the actions of others as negative (Kubzansky et al., 2005; Smith, 1992). Trait hostility increases physiological arousal because of the way hostile people interpret the world; they are more likely to perceive even neutral events as negative, responding strongly because they perceive interpersonal threat (Kiecolt-Glaser & Newton, 2001).

The Health Effects of Hostility

Hostility, like depression, increases the risk of cardiovascular disease, and its effects are additive with other negative emotional states (Smith et al., 2007). Smith and Ruiz's (2002) review noted that people who are high in trait hostility are more prone to ischemia and constriction of the coronary arteries during mental stress. Trait hostility predicted new coronary events in previously healthy people. And for patients who already had coronary heart disease, hostility sped-up progression of the disease.

Hostility also has metabolic effects. In a sample of 1,081 older men, hostility was related to several indices of metabolic syndrome (Niaura et al., 2000). Hostility was positively associated with higher waist/hip ratio, body mass index, total caloric intake, fasting insulin level, and serum triglycerides. It was inversely related to education and HDL cholesterol. The authors concluded that their results were consistent with previous studies indicating that hostility was associated with a pattern of obesity, central adiposity, and elevated insulin levels.

Hostility also increases the risk of metabolic syndrome in teens. In a three year follow-up of 134 white and African American adolescents, hostility at Time 1 predicted risk factors for metabolic syndrome at Time 2 (Raikkonen, Matthews, & Salomon, 2003). These risk factors were at the 75th percentile for age, gender, and race, and included BMI, insulin resistance, a high ratio of triglycerides to HDL cholesterol, and mean arterial blood pressure. Unfortunately, lipid profiles, blood pressure, and insulin resistance are not the only things that hostility affects. Like depression, hostility also increases inflammation.

Hostility and Inflammation

A study of 6,814 healthy men and women found that participants with higher levels of cynical distrust, chronic stress, or depression had higher levels of inflammation (Ranjit et al., 2007). Inflammation included elevated C-reactive protein, IL-6, and fibrinogen. Chronic stress was associated with higher IL-6 and C-reactive protein, and depression was associated with higher IL-6. All are risk factors for heart disease.

Hostility was associated with higher levels of circulating proinflammatory cytokines IL-1α, IL-1ß, and IL-8 in 44 healthy, non-smoking, premenopausal women. The combination of depression and hostility was particularly harmful and increased levels of IL-1ß, IL-8 and TNF-α (Suarez, Lewis, Krishnan, & Young, 2004). There was a dose-response effect: the more severe the depression and hostility, the greater the production of cytokines. A study with men had similar results (Suarez, 2003). The author noted that increased levels of IL-6 predicted both future risk of cardiac events and all-cause mortality. He hypothesized that IL-6 may mediate the relationship between hostility and these health problems.

Suarez (2006) studied 135 healthy patients (75 men, 60 women), with no symptoms of diabetes. He found that women with higher levels of depression and hostility, and who had a propensity to express anger, had higher levels of fasting insulin, glucose, and insulin resistance. These findings were not true for men, and they were independent of other risk factors for metabolic syndrome, including BMI, age, fasting triglycerides, exercise regularity, or ethnicity. The author indicated that these findings were significant since pre-study glucose levels were in the non-diabetic range. The author noted that inflammation, particularly elevated IL-6 and C-reactive protein, may mediate the relationship between depression and hostility, and risk of type-2 diabetes and cardiovascular disease, possibly because they increase insulin resistance.

Marital hostility also increased risk. Women who rated their marriages as unsatisfying had an increased risk of cardiovascular disease over the 13 year marriage (Gallo, Troxel, Matthews, & Kuller 2003). Lack of satisfaction was related to a wide range of cardiovascular risk factors, including low HDL cholesterol and high levels of triglycerides, BMI, blood pressure, depression, and anger.

A three year study of 134 white and African American teens found that hostility at Time 1 predicted at least two risk factors for metabolic syndrome at the 75th percentile for age, gender, and race at Time 2. These risk factors included BMI, insulin resistance, ratio of triglycerides to HDL cholesterol, and arterial blood pressure (Raikkonen et al., 2003).

Hostility also appears to increase the negative impact of depression on health. In a study of 316 older adults, Stewart and colleagues (2008) found that hostility was related to higher levels of C-reactive protein and IL-6 only among people with higher levels of depressive symptoms. The authors noted there were depressive symptoms by hostility interaction for both measures of inflammation.

Summary

Human social relationships either increase or decrease our vulnerability to stress. If humans make consistently negative or hostile appraisals of the motives of others, they increase their risk of disease directly and indirectly by impacting the quality of their social relationships. This vulnerability manifests through several physiological mechanisms, including inflammation. These findings indicate that humans are social animals and that social support, social integration, and perceived social status have measurable effects on health. Indeed, loved ones and others in our social orbit help regulate our internal states. Hostility and disruptions to social networks have a negative impact on health and can result in diseases, such as heart disease, metabolic syndrome, and diabetes.

Posttraumatic Stress Disorder (PTSD)

Trauma survivors are significantly more likely to have a number of serious illnesses and to die prematurely than their non-traumatized counterparts (Felitti et al., 2001; Kendall-Tackett, 2003). For example, the National Comorbidity Study found that women who were maltreated as children had a nine-fold increase in cardiovascular disease compared to non-maltreated women (Batten, Aslan, Maciejewski, & Masure, 2004). Data from the Canadian Community Health Survey (N=36,984) indicated that participants with posttraumatic stress disorder (PTSD) had significantly higher rates of several illnesses, including cardiovascular disease, respiratory diseases, chronic pain syndromes, gastrointestinal illnesses, and cancer (Sareen et al., 2007). PTSD was also strongly associated with chronic fatigue syndrome and multiple-chemical sensitivity, but there was no significant difference in rates of diabetes.

Not surprisingly, people with PTSD use more healthcare services. In a study of women seeking healthcare at Veterans Administration facilities (Dobie et al., 2006), the women with PTSD had more outpatient visits to the emergency department, primary care, medical or surgery subspecialties, ancillary services, and diagnostic tests. They had higher rates of hospitalizations and surgical procedures. Women with PTSD were significantly more likely to have a service-related disability, have chronic pain, and to be obese. They were also more likely to smoke and abuse alcohol. Comorbid depression rates were also high: 75% of the women with PTSD also screened positive for depression.

Inflammation in Trauma Survivors

Although a relatively new area of study, several researchers have found that traumatic events increase levels of proinflammatory cytokines in trauma survivors. The increase in inflammation may mediate the relationship between trauma and health problems.

Childhood maltreatment was shown to affect clinically relevant levels of C-reactive protein when measured 20 years later in abuse survivors (Danese et al., 2007). The participants (N=1,037) were part of the Dunedin Multidisciplinary Health and Development Study, a study of health behavior in a complete birth cohort in New Zealand. Participants were assessed every two to three years throughout childhood, and every five to six years through age 32. The effect of child maltreatment on inflammation was independent of co-occurring life stresses in adulthood, early life risks, or adult health or health behavior. Severity of abuse was related, in a dose-response way, to severity of inflammation.

At the 32-year follow-up of the same cohort, the participants were assessed for the impact of childhood adversity on three age-related disease markers: major depression, high inflammation (C-reactive protein), and a cluster of metabolic risk factors that included overweight, high blood pressure, high cholesterol, low HDL cholesterol, high glycated hemoglobin, and low maximum oxygen consumption (Danese et al., 2009). "Childhood adversity" was defined as low socioeconomic status (SES), child maltreatment, and social isolation. They found that children exposed to childhood adversities were at high risk for all three disease markers. They had elevated risk of depression, high inflammation levels, and high rates of the metabolic risk factors. These risk factors were nonredundant, cumulative, and independent of other risk factors. They noted that childhood adversity has long-term effects on emotional, immune, and metabolic abnormalities.

C-reactive protein was also relevant in another study of PTSD (Spitzer et al., 2010). In this German community sample of 3,049 adults, 55 had diagnoses of PTSD. Participants with PTSD were twice as likely to have C-reactive protein levels higher than 3 mg/L (considered high-risk for cardiovascular disease), even after accounting for other risk factors, such as BMI, blood pressure, lipid profiles, exercise, alcohol, and trauma exposure. The authors note that this is likely one pathway by which PTSD can lead to poor cardiovascular and metabolic health.

In a study of intimate partner violence (IPV), 62 women who had had abusive partners had significantly higher interferon-γ (IFN-γ) levels than non-abused women (Woods et al., 2005). Fifty-two percent of women in the IPV-group reported depression, and 39% had high levels of PTSD symptoms. These findings demonstrated the lingering health effects of intimate partner violence in women who experienced violence eight to 11 years previously, yet were still manifesting significantly physical symptomatology.

Inflammation was also elevated in a study of rape (Groer, Thomas, Evans, Helton, & Weldon, 2006). In this study, 15 women who had been raped were compared with 16 women who had not been sexually assaulted on immune markers 24 to 72 hours after their assault. Women who had been sexually assaulted had higher ACTH, C-reactive protein, IL-6, IL-10, IFN-γ than women in the control group. In addition, the assaulted women had lower B lymphocyte counts and decreased lymphocyte proliferation. The researchers interpreted their findings as indicating that sexual assault activated innate immunity and suppressed some aspects of adaptive immunity. If these long-term alterations persist, they could lead to health problems in rape survivors.

In a sample of 14 otherwise healthy patients with PTSD and a matched group on age and gender of 14 patients without PTSD, von Kanel and colleagues (2006) investigated PTSD and blood coagulation by measuring clotting factors, fibrinogen, and D-dimer in the plasma. They found the more severe the PTSD, the higher the levels of fibrinogen and the clotting factor FVIII:C. They concluded that PTSD may elicit hypercoagulability, even at subthreshold levels, and this may increase the risk for cardiovascular disease in trauma survivors.

Early life adversity has also been shown to increase inflammation in African Americans, in particular. In a study of 177 African Americans and 822 whites (ages=35-86 years), Slopen and colleagues (2010) found that there were significant effects for inflammation for African Americans, but not whites. Early life adversity was measured in three broad categories: stressful events during childhood or adolescent (these included school failure, parental substance abuse or unemployment, and moving two or more times), self-rated relationship with parents, and frequency of verbal or physical assault by parents measured by the Conflicts Tactics Scale. The measures of inflammation they examined were IL-6, fibrinogen, endothelia leukocyte adhesion molecule-1 and soluble intercellular adhesion molecule-1 (sICAM-1). Some of these effects were attenuated by health behaviors, BMI, adult stressors, and depressive symptoms. The authors concluded that early life adversity was predictive of high concentrations of inflammatory markers for midlife African Americans, but not whites.

Sleep Disorders in PTSD

Sleep disorders are common among trauma survivors, with disturbed sleep and nightmares being key symptoms (Morin & Ware, 1996). Sleep problems could be another way that PTSD impacts health (Suarez & Goforth, 2010). A number of studies have documented disturbed sleep patterns in men and women who have experienced a wide range of violence. For example, in a European community sample, 68% of sexual abuse survivors reported having sleep difficulties, with 45% having repetitive nightmares (Teegan, 1999). In a French sample, 33% of teens who had been raped indicated that they "slept badly" compared with 16% of the non-assaulted control group. Of the assaulted teens, 28% had nightmares (compared with 11%), and 56% woke during the night (compared with 21%; Choquet, Darves-Bornoz, Ledoux, Manfredi, & Hassler, 1997).

Hulme (2000) found that sleep problems among female sexual abuse survivors were common in a primary-care sample. Fifty-two percent of sexual abuse survivors reported that they could not sleep at night (compared with 24% of the non-abused group), and 36% reported nightmares (compared with 13%). Intrusive symptoms were also common, with 53% of sexual abuse survivors reporting sudden thoughts or images of past events (compared with 18% of the non-abused group).

In a sample of battered women living in shelters (N=50), 70% reported poor sleep quality, 28% went to bed very fatigued, and 40% woke up feeling very fatigued (Humphreys, Lee, Neylan, & Marmar, 1999). Moreover, 82% described one or more of the following characteristics of disturbed sleep: many wakings over the course of the night, restless sleep, and early-morning waking. Six described vivid nightmares that included recent incidents of abuse.

In a study of sleep disorders in sexual assault survivors, 80% had either sleep-breathing or sleep-movement disorders. Both of these disorders were linked to higher levels of depression and suicidality, and women who had both types of sleep disorders had the most severe symptoms. The authors speculated that fragmented sleep potentiated the symptoms for women after a sexual assault, stretching their fragile coping abilities to the breaking point (Krakow et al., 2000a).

Sleep problems may also keep symptoms of PTSD active. In a study of 23 patients who suffered from chronic nightmares and obstructive sleep apnea, patients who had completed a treatment program for their sleep problems (N=14) were compared with patients who had dropped out of the program (N=9). Twenty-one months later, those who completed the program had substantially improved sleep compared with those who had not. When the patients with PTSD were compared with the PTSD/no-treatment patients, those in the treatment group had 75% improvement in their PTSD symptoms. In contrast, the six patients in the PTSD/no-treatment group reported a 43% worsening of symptoms. The authors concluded that treating sleep difficulties appeared to also improve PTSD symptoms, and recommended a full evaluation of sleep in patients with PTSD (Krakow et al, 2000b).

How Sleep Impacts Health

McEwen (2003) reported that even short periods of sleep deprivation can elevate cortisol and glucose levels, and can increase both insulin and insulin resistance. Sleep deprivation also provokes an inflammatory response since the body thinks it's under attack. Long-term sleep deprivation can seriously impair health, and this could be a health risk factor for men and women who are not in stable, secure relationships (Stein, Belik, Jacobi, & Sareen, 2008). Suarez and Goforth (2010) note that sleep disorders, such as primary insomnia and obstructive sleep apnea, increase inflammatory markers, such as C-reactive protein, IL-6, and TNF-α. Subclinical sleep disorders increase the risk of cardiovascular disease, type-2 diabetes, metabolic syndrome, and all-cause mortality.

A meta-analysis of sleep duration and obesity of 36 studies that included 634,511 children and adults found that short sleep duration (< 5 hours) is related to obesity worldwide (Cappuccio et al., 2008). A large study of snoring and witnessed sleep apnea in a general population study of 7,905 men and women (aged 25-79 years) in Sweden found that snoring and witnessed sleep apnea was related to diabetes mellitus in women (Valham et al., 2009). This effect was independent of smoking, age, BMI, or waist circumference. This relationship was not true for men.

Sleep problems also increase the risk of depression. In a general population study in Japan (N=24,686), adults who slept less than six hours or more than eight had the highest rates of depression. Those who slept between six to eight hours had the lowest rates of all (Kaneita, Uchiyama, Yoshiike, & Ohida, 2006). In a sample of new mothers, those who sleep less than four hours between midnight and 6 a.m., and who had daytime naps of less than 60 minutes had the highest rates of depression at three months (Goyal, Gay, & Lee, 2009). The strongest predictors of depression were problems falling asleep and excessive daytime sleepiness.

Another study of 1,666 men and 2,329 women in Japan found that for women, both short and long sleep durations are associated with high serum triglyceride levels and low HDL cholesterol (Kaneita et al., 2008). The strongest effects were found for women sleeping five hours or less per night. The authors concluded that usual sleep duration was closely associated with lipid and lipoprotein levels.

A study with an American sample had similar findings (Hall et al., 2008). This study included 1,214 participants. They found that sleep of short and long duration increased the risk of metabolic syndrome more than 45% compared with those sleeping seven to eight hours a night. Sleep duration was also individually associated with several symptoms of metabolic syndrome, including abdominal obesity, elevated fasting glucose, and hypertriglyceridemia.

How Breastfeeding Protects Women's Health

Breastfeeding Downregulates the Stress Response

A recent review found that rates of depression are lower in breastfeeding mothers than their non-breastfeeding counterparts (Dennis & McQueen, 2009). As described earlier, breastfeeding protects maternal mental health because it downregulates the stress response. This downregulation confers a survival advantage by protecting the breastfeeding mother and directing her toward milk production, conservation of energy, and nurturing behaviors (Groer, Davis, & Hemphill, 2002). Hormones related to lactation, such as oxytocin and prolactin, have both antidepressant and anxiolytic effects (Sibolboro Mezzacappa & Endicott, 2007).

Breastfeeding's downregulation of the stress response explains the recent findings regarding cardiovascular disease (Schwartz et al., 2009). This study included 139,681 postmenopausal women described in the introduction. The researchers found lower cardiovascular risk for breastfeeding women compared to those who never breastfed: the longer women lactated, the lower their cardiovascular risk. The authors noted that lactation improves glucose tolerance, lipid metabolism, and C-reactive protein.

Another study found that breastfeeding was related to lower C-reactive protein, another inflammatory marker for cardiovascular and other chronic diseases, in 26-year-old women who participated in the Dunedin Multidisciplinary Health Study (Williams, Williams, & Poulton, 2006).

Breastfeeding Alters Metabolism

Lactation may also lower the risk of metabolic and cardiovascular disease because of its changes in metabolism. A number of theories have been offered. Ram et al. (2008) argue that lactation creates a "metabolic drain" that alters energy homeostasis. It increases HDL levels, decreases triglycerides, and improves insulin sensitivity, making the body a more "energy-efficient machine."

Stuebe and Rich-Edwards (2009) describe the "reset hypothesis." During gestation, visceral fat accumulates, insulin resistance increases, and both lipid and triglyceride levels increase. Breastfeeding helps reverse–or reset–these changes. For maternal metabolism, pregnancy ends with weaning, not birth.

Breastfeeding Mothers Get More Sleep

Breastfeeding mothers also get more sleep, and this too could protect their long-term health. In a study of 33 mothers at four weeks postpartum, Quillin and Glenn (2004) found that mothers who were breastfeeding slept more than mothers who were bottle-feeding. Data were collected via questionnaire that recorded five days of mother and newborn sleep. When comparing whether bedsharing made a difference in total sleep, they found that bedsharing, breastfeeding mothers got the most sleep, and breastfeeding mothers who were not bedsharing got the least amount of sleep. Mothers who were bottle-feeding got the same amount of sleep whether their babies were with them or in another room.

Sleep patterns of 72 couples were compared from pregnancy to the first month postpartum via sleep diaries and wrist actigraphy (Gay, Lee, & Lee, 2004). Most of the mothers were at least partially breastfeeding (94%), and 80% were exclusively breastfeeding. Most of the babies slept in their parents' room, and 51% regularly slept in their parents' beds. Sleep and fatigue outcomes were not associated with type of birth, parent-infant bedsharing, or baby's age. Mothers who were exclusively breastfeeding had a greater number of nighttime wakings (30 vs. 24) compared with mothers who were not breastfeeding exclusively. The exclusively breastfeeding mothers slept approximately 20 minutes longer than mothers not exclusively breastfeeding.

A study from France compared fatigue levels in exclusively breastfeeding (N=129) and exclusively formula-feeding mothers (N=114) at two to four days, six and 12 weeks postpartum (Callahan, Sejourne, &

Denis, 2006). They found no significant difference between the groups at any time point on the measure of maternal fatigue. The authors suggested that all mothers experience postpartum fatigue, independent of feeding method, and informing mothers ahead of time that breastfeeding is not likely the cause of their fatigue may help them persist.

In a study of mothers and fathers at three months postpartum, data were collected via wrist actigraphy and using sleep diaries (Doan, Gardiner, Gay, & Lee, 2007). The study compared sleep of exclusively breastfed infants vs. those supplemented with formula. In this sample, 67% were fed exclusively with breast milk, 23% were fed a combination of breast milk and formula, and 10% were exclusively formula fed. Mothers who exclusively breastfed slept an average of 40 minutes longer than mothers who supplemented. Parents of infants who were breastfed during the night slept an average of 40 to 45 minutes more than parents of infants given formula. Parents of formula-fed infants had more sleep disturbances. They concluded that parents who are supplementing with formula under the assumption that they are going to get more sleep should be encouraged to breastfeed, so they will get an extra 30-40 minutes of sleep per night.

Not only do breastfeeding mothers get more sleep, but their sleep appears to be better quality. Blyton, Sullivan & Edwards (2002) compared 12 exclusively breastfeeding women, 12 age-matched control women, and seven women who were exclusively bottlefeeding. They found that total sleep time and REM sleep time were similar in the three groups of women. The marked difference between the groups was in the amount of slow-wave sleep (SWS). The breastfeeding mothers got an average of 182 minutes of SWS. Women in the control group had an average of 86 minutes. And the exclusively bottle-feeding women had an average of 63 minutes. Among the breastfeeding women, there was a compensatory reduction in light, non-REM sleep.

In another study, poor sleep was an independent risk factor for depression. Among the factors associated with poor sleep was "not exclusively breastfeeding." This was a risk factor for both sleep problems and postpartum depression in a study of 2,830 women at seven weeks postpartum (Dorheim, Bondevik, Eberhard-Gran, & Bjorvatn, 2009).

Kendall-Tackett, Cong, and Hale's (2011) recent study found that breastfeeding mothers reported more total hours of sleep than their mixed- or formula-feeding counterparts. These findings were from the Survey of Mothers' Sleep and Fatigue that included 6,410 mothers of infants 0-12 months worldwide. Breastfeeding mothers reported significantly less daily fatigue, more energy, and higher levels of physical well-being than mixed-

or formula-feeding mothers. Mixed- and formula-feeding mothers were not significantly different from each other on all measures.

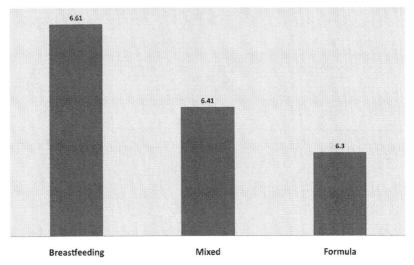

$F(2)=15.55, p<.0001$

Figure 5-1. Breastfeeding mothers report significantly more sleep than mixed- or formula-feeding mothers. From Kendall-Tackett, Cong, & Hale, (2011, in press). Used with permission.

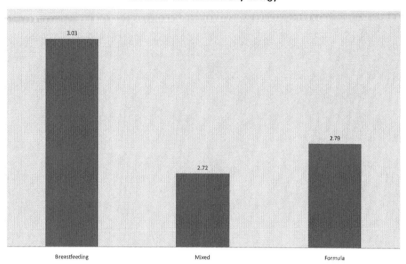

$F(2)=46.9, p<.0001$
Figure 5-2. Breastfeeding mothers report significantly higher daily energy levels than mixed- or formula-feeding mothers. From Kendall-Tackett, Cong, & Hale (2011). Used with permission.

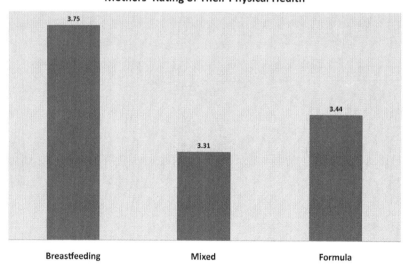

$F(2)=78.03, p<.0001$
Figure 5-3. Breastfeeding mothers rate their physical health as better than mixed- or formula-feeding mothers. From Kendall-Tackett, Cong, & Hale (2011, in press). Used with permission.

Depressed mood, anhedonia, and overall score on the Patient Health Questionnaire-2 (a measure of depression) were significantly lower for breastfeeding mothers than the other two groups. Mixed-feeding mothers did not significantly differ from formula-feeding mothers on all depression measures, suggesting that breastfeeding was a qualitatively different experience than mixed- or formula-feeding, and was more protective of maternal mental health.

Feeling Down, Depressed or Hopeless

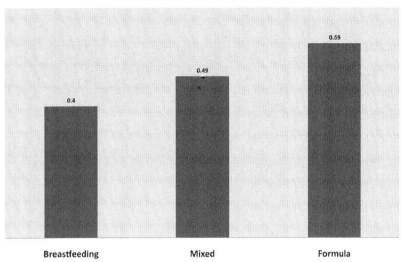

$F(2)=13.53, p<.0001$

Figure 5-4. Breastfeeding mothers are significantly less likely to report depressed mood than mixed- or formula-feeding mothers. From Kendall-Tackett, Cong, & Hale (2011, in press). Used with permission.

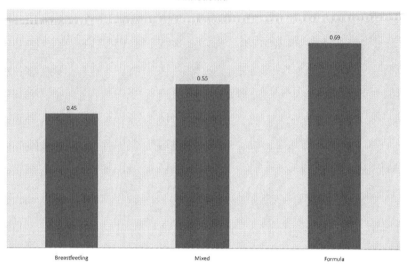

$F(2)=13.27$, $p<.0001$

Figure 5-5. Breastfeeding mothers are significantly less likely to report anhedonia. From Kendall-Tackett, Cong, & Hale (2011, in press).

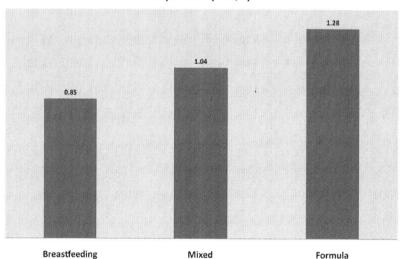

$F(2)=17.23$, $p<.0001$

Figure 5-6. Breastfeeding mothers are significantly less likely to report depression on the PHQ-2 than mixed- or formula-feeding mothers. From Kendall-Tackett, Cong, & Hale (2011, in press). Used with permission.

Breastfeeding and Hostility

There is no specific study of general hostility related to feeding method. But there is a good proxy for one: a study examining the effects of breastfeeding on maternal-perpetrated child maltreatment. This was a 15 year cohort study of 7,223 Australian mother-infant pairs (Strathearn, Mamun, Najman, O'Callaghan, 2009). In this sample, there were 512 substantiated reports of child maltreatment, which was 4.3% of the cohort. Breastfeeding decreased the risk of maternal-perpetrated child maltreatment. Mothers were 2.6 times more likely to abuse their children if they were not breastfeeding. The results for child neglect were even more striking. Risk of neglect decreased as breastfeeding duration increased. Non-breastfeeding mothers were 3.8 times more likely to neglect their children compared with mothers who breastfed for more than four months. If mothers breastfed for less than four months, they were 2.3 times more likely to neglect their children compared with mothers who breastfeed longer than four months. The authors speculated that the abuse-lowering effects of breastfeeding may be due to oxytocin, which reduces anxiety, elevates mood, increases maternal responsiveness, lowers maternal stress, and increases attachment.

Breastfeeding seems to have a similar long-term positive effect on the children as well. In a 14-year longitudinal study from Western Australia, a cohort of pregnant women and their children were assessed at two, six, eight, ten, and 14 years (Oddy et al., 2009). Longer duration of breastfeeding was associated with better child mental health, assessed by the Child Behavior Checklist (CBCL), at every assessment point. There appeared a dose-response effect: the longer the children were breastfed, the better their mental health. For example, at age two, CBCL average score for children never breastfed was 16.1 vs. 9.6 for children breastfed for at least 12 months (lower scores mean less pathology). Similarly, at age five the average score for never breastfed was 26.3 vs. 16 for children breastfed at least 12 months. At age eight, the scores were 19.2 vs. 13.5. At age ten, they were 15.2 vs. 12.6, and at age 14, they were 16.7 vs. 10.9.

Conclusions

Several recent large studies have found that breastfeeding, particularly 12 months or longer, confers women lifetime protection against cardiovascular and metabolic disease. This chapter has summarized studies that suggest several possible mechanisms for how breastfeeding protects women's lifetime health. Breastfeeding downregulates the stress and inflammatory response system, lowers the risk of depression and hostility, and increases the mother-infant bond. It also improves sleep quality by increasing the total number of sleep hours and improving mothers' overall sense of physical well-being during the postpartum period. From these studies, we can conclude that breastfeeding–particularly exclusive breastfeeding–protects women's physical and mental well-being. And the good news is that these effects persist long past the perinatal period.

Chapter 6. Breastfeeding and Immunity

Maternal health appears to be favored in women who have breastfed. Or to turn the phrase, formula feeding increases health risks. There are both early and later effects on health that have been studied.

Early Effects

Enteromammary Link

Lactation requires an enormous amount of regulation, not only in the production and letdown of milk, but also in the multiple pathways involved in the immune composition of milk. The homing of cells from the common mucosal system to the breast, with the resultant production of many cytokines, chemokines, and growth factors, is extraordinarily effective and complex. Known as the enteromammary link, T and B lymphocytes that are responsive to maternal gastrointestinal antigens, migrate to the breast in late pregnancy, and begin to secrete Immunoglobulin A (IgA) dimers that ultimately attach to secretory factor and produce sIgA. This sIgA is specific to maternal antigens and is secreted into the milk, and protects the breastfeeding infant from the common antigens the infant is exposed to by contact with its mother. This contact is during birth and produces a population of bacteria almost instantly in the infant that are the maternal microbiota (Hanson & Korotkova, 2002). Breastmilk sIgA is present in amounts of 0.5 g per day. Once virgin cells are committed, they express "homing" receptors that are specific for distant mucosal sites and "migrate" to the breast and other glands. It is in the local environment of the breast and in the milk itself that B cell secretion of sIgA occurs. This important and understudied pathway is depicted in Figure 6-1.

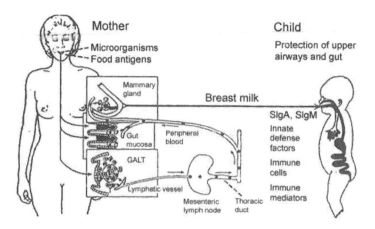

Figure 6-1. The enteromammary link. From Brandtzaeg, 1998. Used with permission.

There are other common mucosal–mammary links, such as the bronchomammary link. The cells which have "homed" to the mammary gland also travel into the milk where they continue to secrete sIgA. Lymphocytes also secrete cytokines, chemokines, and growth factors in the milk, which are important defense molecules to protect and mature the neonatal gut. While clearly the goal of these links is to protect the infant, maternal physiology plays an essential part, and the maternal immune system must be competent in order to carry out these complex processes. Evolution has dictated that the major protection of the neonate is through its mother, and thus it is likely that mothers are protected in the postpartum period.

Health and Immunity in the Early Postpartum

Groer studied health and immunity in postpartum mothers, measured between four and six weeks after birth (Groer et al., 2005). The mean age of the mothers in the study was 26 years. They were 88% Caucasian, 1% Asian, 6% African American, 3% Hispanic; 66% were married; one quarter had income levels below $25,000; and one quarter had income levels greater than $40,000. There were 183 postpartum mothers who had uncomplicated pregnancy and birth histories. Ninety-nine were exclusively breastfeeding, and 84 were exclusively formula feeding. In addition, 33 age and income matched controls were studied. Our research suggests that postpartum mothers, in general, have a somewhat upregulated inflammatory response system compared to control women as depicted in Figures 6-2 and 6-3.

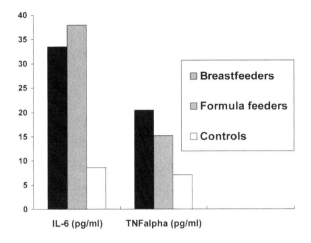

Figure 6-2. Inflammatory cytokines.

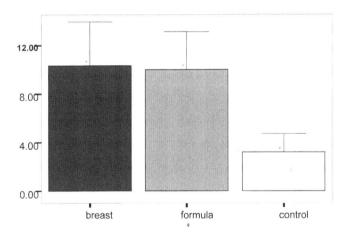

Figure 6-3. C-reactive protein.

Figure 6-2 shows a significant difference in interleukin-6 (IL-6), and tumor necrosis factor-α (TNF-α) in postpartum mothers compared to controls. These are pro inflammatory cytokines that are normally released in responses to threats, such as microbial infection. Levels of C-reactive protein (CRP) are also very high (Figure 6-3). CRP is released in response to IL-6 by the liver and acts to perpetuate an inflammatory state. So the postpartum state measured at this point in time has an appropriate degree of proinflammatory protection as the maternal immune system recovers from the immunosuppression of pregnancy. This state is actually very similar to what happens to the immune system in pregnancy. Does the upregulated inflammatory process signal a kind of alerted innate immune system immediately tagging and killing microorganisms that pose a threat to the maternal-infant dyad? Taking an evolutionary perspective may be helpful. Certainly, the maternal-infant immunological dyadic relationships evolved in a far different environment than that which is now common in Western societies. Infants are born essentially sterile, but very quickly become colonized with maternal gut flora, beginning at delivery. Milk provides appropriate antibodies to maternal gut colonizers to which the infant is likely exposed, but production of antibodies is an energy requiring process for mothers. Exposure of the infant to large doses of multiple bacterial strains is a threat, and the maternal enteromammeric link must keep up with this threat to protect her nursing infant. So it makes some sense that a postpartum mother would elaborate many defenses to protect the dyad from infection, with secretion of Immunoglobulin A into the milk if the microbes become established in her flora. This could include an upregulated innate immune system. Of course, too much inflammation would end up being detrimental, and breastfeeders differ from formula feeders in the amount of inflammation present. We have found that over the first six months of the postpartum, breastfeeders have consistently lower IL-6 levels in their plasma compared to formula feeders. This is true for both exclusive and partial breastfeeders.

Is there a differential health benefit conferred by differences in immune responses in breast compared to formula feeding mothers? We have reported that postpartum mothers have significantly fewer common infection symptoms, report less common health problems, and take fewer prescription medications than controls. And we have suggested that the immune and inflammatory characteristics of the postpartum might be protective. Figures 6-4 to 6-8 show the differences between formula feeders compared to exclusively breastfeeding mothers, measured cross-sectionally between four and six weeks postpartum. The mothers were asked to complete the Carr Infection Symptom Checklist, which allows for both frequency and severity of symptoms of common infections to be recorded. Mothers were asked to record symptoms they had experienced since the birth of their baby. They were told not to include symptoms that they were sure were related to allergy. In Figures 6-4, 6-5, 6-6, and 6-7, the various categories of symptoms are depicted, showing in nearly every case breastfeeding women reported fewer incidences of these symptoms.

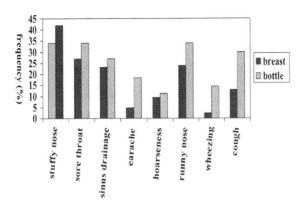

Figure 6-4. Respiratory symptoms.

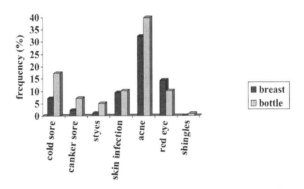

Figure 6-5. Skin and eye symptoms.

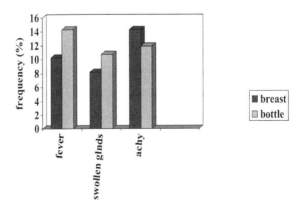

Figure 6-6. Flu symptoms.

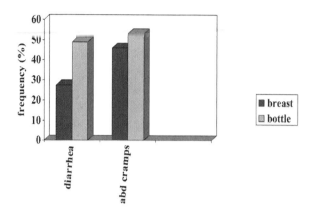

Figure 6-7. Gastrointestinal symptoms.

In Figure 6-8, there is evidence that breastfeeding women had more frequent incidences of vaginal and genitourinary symptoms. In this case, the risk might be related to the lower estrogen and progesterone levels associated with breastfeeding.

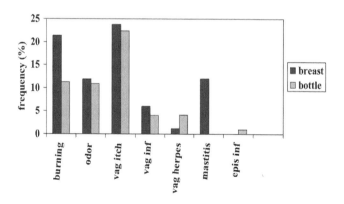

Figure 6-8. Reproductive/urinary tract symptoms.

This health benefit is seen when factors that might influence infection risk are controlled, such as income, marital status, and even smoking, although few of the breastfeeding women smoked.

The lower frequency and severities of symptoms of infectious illnesses reported by exclusively lactating women suggest a significant health protection of these mothers. Perhaps there is an evolutionary benefit for health in postpartum mothers that is related to innate immune activation. It is important to realize that humans are the only animal species that chooses not to lactate. When we compare animal studies to human conditions, this point is not always apparent. Postnatal animal mothers are always lactating! Animal research suggests that the postnatal period is a health-protected state. Wound healing was accelerated in lactating rats compared to controls, and there was a differential expression of proinflammatory cytokines and chemokines in the wounded tissue compared to non-lactating controls (Detillion et al., 2003). Oxytocin applied to wounds in Siberian hamsters lowered stress-induced cortisol concentrations compared to vehicle treated animals, and decreased wound size at several time points (Detillion, Craft, Glasper, Prendergast, & DeVries, 2004). We have reported that milk secretory IgA is elevated in mothers who have more antigenic exposure, suggesting a responsive mucosal immune system (Groer, Davis, & Steele, 2004). Are there perhaps physiological mechanisms by which postpartum mothers (and their infants) are protected from infection and have generally good health?

A report of health in a large cohort of women in San Francisco suggested that physical health improved in the postpartum compared to pregnancy. Lack of exercise and poverty were associated with poor health in these women, both during and after pregnancy (Haas et al., 2005). A prospective study of 261 expectant fathers and mothers during pregnancy and at six months postpartum regarding health, partner, and work characteristics indicated that mothers experienced an increase in vitality despite sleep deficits (Gjerdingen & Center, 2003).

The largest study of postpartum health seems to be one carried out in 1993 in Victoria, Australia. This study surveyed health problems in 1,336 mothers and found that nearly 12% of the total sample indicated more coughs or colds than usual during the first six months, compared to normal (Brown & Lumley, 1998). These data are subjective. Endometritis is the most common postpartum infection. Other infections include: 1) postsurgical wound infections, 2) perineal cellulitis, 3) mastitis, 4) respiratory complications from anesthesia, 5) retained products of conception, 6) urinary tract infections (UTIs), and 7) septic pelvic phlebitis (Wong & Rosh, 2010). These are all fairly serious, but early infections. Yet the incidence is low, and the mortality rate is 0.6 maternal deaths per 100,000 live births. Most studies of infection have examined the very early postpartum period, and there has been a focus on HIV disease in the literature. Only a few studies, including ours, have looked at common (mostly viral) infections, and all are flawed by the self-report nature of the collected data and lack of attention to confounders that could influence health.

In Groer's studies, we have found evidence that there is greater capacity for stimulated lymphocyte proliferation in breastfeeding women compared to formula-feeding women and controls. Figure 6-9 shows experiments in which lymphocytes from exclusively breastfeeding women were compared to those from formula-feeding women. Cells were stimulated by powerful mitogens (PHA and ConA) in culture for five days, and then radioactive thymidine was added to the cultures. The thymidine becomes incorporated into the DNA of the cells and is a marker of mitotic activity of the cells. The results are computed as the stimulation index (S.I.). The breastfeeders had a much more proliferative response, indicating a more active population of T cells, compared to formula feeders or controls.

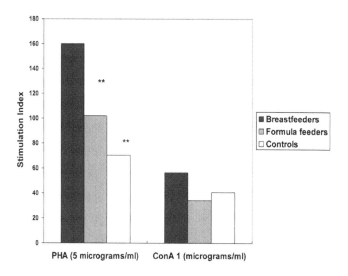

Figure 6-9. Stimulation index.

Weight Loss

Exclusively breastfeeding women often achieve their pre-pregnancy weights about six months earlier than women who exclusively bottle-fed their infants. Many older studies suggest that weight loss in exclusively breastfeeding women is related to use of pregnancy fat reserves that can provide metabolic energy for milk production. On the other hand, many lactating women report increased caloric intake, so weight loss may not universally occur. It is not advisable for lactating women to exercise heavily in the early postpartum. We found a pattern of proinflammatory cytokines, which were increased in heavily exercising, exclusively lactating women (Groer & Shelton, 2009). This suggested that these cytokines, which normally are very low in concentration in human milk, represented a danger signal to the infant gut.

Lifelong Benefits of Breastfeeding

Evidence suggests that breastfeeding mothers are in many ways protected from acute and chronic health problems. Of course, the duration and exclusivity of the breastfeeding periods in a mother's life are likely to be important in these relationships. Most of these beneficial effects are achieved when breastfeeding has had a duration of at least six months and has been exclusive during that time.

Type-2 Diabetes

As described in the introduction and Chapter 5, there is accumulating evidence that breastfeeding protects mothers from later development of type-2 diabetes. This may be related to metabolic changes and programming that occurs during lactation, which reduces risk. In animal studies, lactation appears to increase insulin sensitivity (Burnol, Guerre-Millo, Lavau, & Girard, 1986). Data from human studies with large samples have shown similar effects (Schwartz et al., 2009). Moreover, this is a dose-respone effect: the longer the duration of lactation, the lower the risk of disease.

Autoimmune Disease

Breastfeeding is known to suppress the HPA response to stress. Researchers (Lankarani-Fard, Kritz-Silverstein, Barrett-Connor, & Goodman-Gruen, 2001) found that this effect may last for years, in that, middle-aged women who had breastfed had higher cortisol levels, and the more pregnancies, the higher the cortisol. Since cortisol is anti-inflammatory, it is possible that breastfeeding may protect against autoimmune diseases, but there are few studies.

Cardiovascular Disease (CVD)

As described earlier, Schwarz et al. (2009) examined the influence of lactation on cardiovascular disease (CVD). Lactation again conferred a protective effect, in that hypertension incidence was lower, as was hyperlipidemia and CVD. These women were not less likely to be obese. The protective effect was seen in women with 12 or more months of lactation.

In a study of aortic and coronary calcification in women age 45-58 years who had breastfed compared to mothers who had not, there was significantly more calcification and plaque, suggesting that vascular changes associated with cardiovascular disease are increased in mothers who do not breastfeed (Schwarz et al., 2010).

Breast and Ovarian Cancer

Most studies do not distinguish between exclusive and partial breastfeeding. All studies reported a statistically significant reduced risk or odds of breast cancer with increased duration of breastfeeding, which varied across the studies (Ip et al., 2007). The biology underlying a protective effect of breastfeeding on breast cancer risk is not understood. Studies suggest decreased risk of breast cancer in women with a lifetime breastfeeding of greater than 12 months. This seems to be true for premenopausal women. Possible mechanisms include hormonal changes (including reduced estrogen), removal of estrogens through milk, excretion of carcinogens through breastfeeding, full differentiation of mammary epithelial cells, and delay of ovulation (Lipworth, Bailey, & Trichopoulos, 2000).

Cumulative breastfeeding for less than 12 months was not statistically significantly associated with a decreased risk of ovarian cancer in a meta-analysis of six studies, including 1,911 cases and 5,007 controls in total (ORadj 0.95; 95%CI: 0.80 – 1.12; Ip et al., 2007). Breastfeeding of at least 12 months cumulative duration was associated with 28% lower odds for ovarian cancer.

Osteoporosis

Intuitively one would expect that long periods of breastfeeding would result in calcium deficits, which would lead to osteopenia and osteoporosis. While there is some bone loss during the period of lactation, there is compensation for it, and breastfeeding has no deleterious effects on bone health (Hadji et al., 2002). In reality, some studies even suggest a beneficial effect of lactation on the incidence of osteoporosis in later life.

Conclusion

Breastfeeding is the natural, normal way of feeding infants. Benefits to the mothers are apparent in short-term effects, such as family planning, decreased infections, and weight loss. Long-term effects, which ultimately would determine quality of life and longevity, are also apparent and significant. These health effects include diabetes, cardiovascular disease, and reproductive cancers. Most breastfeeding mothers are unaware of any personal health benefits of lactation, and it may be information that would help them sustain breastfeeding for longer periods of time.

Chapter 7. The Implications of an Anti-Inflammatory Approach to Enhancing the Health Effects of Breastfeeding throughout Women's Lives

As we described in Chapter 5, depression and other negative mental states not only create misery for those who suffer from them, these mental states also increase the risk for physical disease. The line between mental and physical illness continues to be blurred. And in fact, researchers are increasingly recognizing that human beings are "mind-bodies," and that what affects one will likely impact the other.

Nowhere is this relationship more aptly demonstrated than in the research on treatments for depression. Maes and colleagues (2009) explain that current theories of depression, particularly serotonergic dysfunction and cortisol hypersecretion, do not provide sufficient explanation for the nature of depression, and treatments that target either of these symptoms are only partially successful. However, a now large body of literature supports the inflammatory etiology of depression. In addition, heart disease, metabolic syndrome, diabetes, cancer, MS, and Alzheimer's all appear to have an inflammatory etiology (Robles, Glaser, & Kiecolt-Glaser, 2005). Recent research suggests that all effective treatments for depression lower inflammation.

This new research on depression suggests it has implications substantially above and beyond simply addressing a mental health issue. Indeed, it suggests that a key to long-term health is downregulating the stress system, particularly the actions of the inflammatory response system. Breastfeeding is one important component in helping women downregulate stress. Other modalities can also help in not only lowering depression, but in lowering women's risk of other inflammatory conditions and diseases throughout their lives. Below is a brief summary of some of this recent research on Omega-3 fatty acids, exercise, psychotherapy, St. John's wort, and antidepressants.

Omega-3 Fatty Acids and Women's Health

Omega-3 fatty acids are specifically anti-inflammatory, and this characteristic helps them both prevent and treat depression, cardiovascular disease, and other inflammatory conditions (Kendall-Tackett, 2007a, 2007b, 2010a, 2010b, 2011; Mischoulon, 2009; Su, 2009). With regard to inflammatory disorders, it is the long-chain Omega-3s that are of interest: eicosapentaenoic acid (EPA) and docosahexaenoic acid (DHA). Humans do not efficiently synthesize these fatty acids and need to consume them directly (Su, 2009).

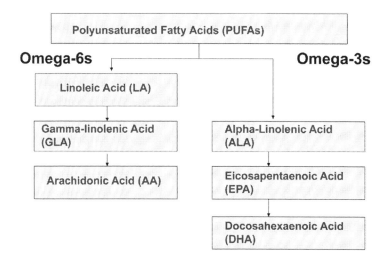

Wang et al. Agency for Healthcare Research & Quality, 2004

Figure 7-1. Comparison of Omega-6 vs Omega-3 fatty acids. From Wang et al., 2004. Used with permission.

Alpha-linolenic acid (ALA) is the parent Omega-3 fatty acid and is found in plant sources. ALA is metabolically too far removed from EPA and DHA to be sufficiently anti-inflammatory, meaning that Omega-3s found in flax seed, walnuts, and other plant sources cannot be used to prevent or treat depression (Freeman et al., 2006; Kendall-Tackett, 2010b). Fish and fish-oil products continue to be the only source of EPA and a good source of DHA (vegetarian DHA products are also available). Unfortunately, in many Western cultures, women tend to consume small amounts Omega-3 fatty acids in their diets and consume too many proinflammatory Omega-6s (Kendall-Tackett, 2011).

Omega-6s and Omega-3s are both polyunsaturated fatty acids (PUFAs). Omega-6s are proinflammatory and are found in vegetable oils, such as corn and safflower oils. Omega-6s are necessary for good nutrition. But they become harmful when they are too abundant in the diet (Mischoulon, 2009). Kiecolt-Glaser and colleagues (2007) noted that the hunter-gatherer diet had an estimated ratio of Omega-6s:Omega-3s of 2:1 or 3:1. In contrast, the typical ratio in the North American diet is approximately 17:1. This dramatic shift corresponds to an upsurge in a number of inflammatory disorders over the past 100 years, including depression, heart disease, and metabolic syndrome. Chronic deficiencies of EPA and DHA increase the risk for disease throughout the lifespan, but the puerperal period appears to be a time of heightened vulnerability (Kendall-Tackett, 2010a; Kiecolt-Glaser et al., 2007; Maes et al., 2009; Su, 2009). Because babies specifically need DHA in particular for brain and vision development, women's bodies will preferentially divert it to their babies. With each subsequent pregnancy, women are further depleted (Rees, Austin, & Parker, 2005).

Stress, Inflammation, and Omega-3s

EPA lowers inflammation by competing for the same metabolic pathways as proinflammatory arachidonic acid. When EPA is present, it blocks arachidonic acid and thereby halts the arachidonic cascade, which leads to the synthesis of prostaglandins, leukotrienes, and eicosanoids (Su, 2009). A recent review found that people with major depression had significantly higher ratios of arachidonic acid to EPA in both serum cholesteryl esters and phospholipids (Parker et al., 2006). In a large population study, high levels of Omega-3s (ALA, EPA, and DHA) in participants' plasma were related to lower levels of the proinflammatory cytokines IL-1α, IL-1ß, IL-6, and TNF-α. For people with low levels of Omega-3s, the opposite was true (Ferrucci et al., 2006).

EPA and DHA also appear to downregulate the stress response (Kendall-Tackett, 2007a). In a study of college students, those deficient in EPA/DHA had a heightened inflammatory response to lab-induced stressors. In contrast, students with higher levels of EPA/DHA were more resilient to stress and had a lower inflammatory response to stress (Maes, Christophe, Bosmans, Lin, & Neels, 2000). A study from Japan had similar findings (Hamazaki et al., 2005). In a double-blind trial, participants took either a placebo or 762 mg of EPA/DHA for two months. The researchers noted that EPA concentrations increased in the red blood cell membranes of the supplemented group. The EPA/DHA group also had significantly decreased levels of plasma norepinephrine.

Kiecolt-Glaser and colleagues (2007), in their study of 43 older adults, noted that prior episodes of stress and depression appeared to "prime" the inflammatory response, making individuals more susceptible to subsequent stress. Even modest supplementation with EPA and DHA, however, lowered levels of norepinephrine, indicating an attenuated stress response. Because of these downregulatory effects on the stress system, EPA and DHA might also have efficacy in the treatment of posttraumatic stress disorder (Kendall-Tackett, 2009). Patients with PTSD often have stress systems that are hyperresponsive to stress. Being replete in EPA and DHA may attenuate their response to future stressors.

Exercise

Exercise has a long track record as a preventative intervention and treatment for metabolic syndrome, diabetes, and heart disease. It has only been recently used as a treatment for depression. Traditionally, exercise has been recommended for people with mild-to-moderate depression. But as two clinical trials have found, exercise can also alleviate major depression as effectively as medications. In the first trial, depressed older adults were randomly assigned to one of three groups: exercise alone, sertraline alone, or a combination of exercise and sertraline (Babyak et al., 2000). After four months of intervention, all the patients improved. Most importantly, there were no differences between the groups: exercise went head-to-head with Zoloft and was as effective in treating depression. People in the exercise-only group did as well as people in the two medication groups. In addition, people in the exercise-only group were significantly less likely to relapse. Six months after completion of treatment, 28% of the exercise-only group became depressed again vs. 51% of the medications-only and medications-exercise groups. The authors concluded that exercise is an effective intervention, even in patients with major depression.

This same group of researchers replicated their findings with another sample (Blumenthal et al., 2007). In the more recent study, 202 adults with major depression were randomized to one of four conditions: sertraline, exercise at home, supervised exercise, or a placebo control. After four months of treatment, 41% of the total sample was in remission, meaning that they no longer met the criteria for major depression. Efficacy rates by treatment were as follows: supervised exercise=45%, home-based exercise=40%, medication=47%, and placebo=31%. Participants in the exercise group walked for 45 minutes on a treadmill at 70% to 85% maximum heart rate capacity, three times a week for 16 weeks. The home-exercise group received the same instructions, but exercised at home, and was therefore not supervised and had minimal contact with the research staff. The authors concluded that the efficacy of exercise was comparable to medications. The supervised program was especially effective, but the home program was also comparable to medications. And all treatments were more effective than the placebo.

Exercise and Inflammation

As the above-cited studies indicate, exercise is an effective treatment for depression. Several psychosocial explanations have been offered for these effects, including increased social connections, improved perceptions of fitness, and improved self-efficacy (McAuley, Blissmer, Katula, Duncan, & Mihalko, 2000). More recently, researchers also found that exercise lowers inflammation. Initially, exercise acts as an acute physical stressor and raises IL-6 and TNF-α. An initial burst of these cytokines does not appear to be harmful. Indeed, and as Goebel and colleagues (2000) point out, in a normally functioning system, high levels of cytokines trigger the body's anti-inflammatory mechanisms to keep inflammation in check.

Over a longer period of time, however, especially in people with chronically elevated proinflammatory cytokines, exercise lowers inflammation. As was true for exercise studies in general, the anti-inflammatory effects of exercise have been studied frequently with older adults. Levels of proinflammatory cytokines naturally increase as people age. Indeed, researchers hypothesize that this age-related rise in inflammation creates vulnerability to diseases, such as heart disease, cancer, and Alzheimer's (Kiecolt-Glaser et al., 2007). Because of this increased vulnerability of older adults to chronic disease, they are frequently the population of choice for studies on exercise, depression, and inflammation.

A study of adults, ages 60 to 90, tested the effect of physical activity on perceived stress, mood, and quality of life, and serum IL-6 and cortisol. The exercise group (N=10) was instructed to walk for 30 minutes, at a rate that would elevate their heart rate to 60% of its maximal capacity, five times a week for the ten-week study. Adults in the control group (N=10) did not engage in physical activity. After the ten-week exercise intervention, the exercise group had significantly lower stress on the Perceived Stress Scale, and improved mood and quality of life on the SF-36 Health Questionnaire. They reported better physical functioning, more vitality, better mental health, and less bodily pain. They also had a significant decrease in serum IL-6 (Starkweather, 2007). Depression did not mediate these findings; this effect was independent of an association between psychological variables and IL-6.

Another study of older adults compared cardio workouts to flexibility/ resistance training to see if either type lowered inflammation (Kohut et al., 2006). In this study, 83 adults, ages 64 to 87, were randomized to one of the two conditions. The cardio workouts were 45 minutes, at 60% to 80% of maximal cardiac effort, three times a week for ten months. The flexibility/resistance workouts were 45 minutes of resistance and flexibility training, three times a week, also for ten months. Both types of exercise led to improved levels of depression, optimism, and sense of coherence. At the end of ten months, the cardio workout had a stronger effect on inflammation. The cardio workout significantly reduced C-reactive protein, IL-6, and IL-18. TNF-α levels improved with both cardio and flexibility/ resistance program. These effects were independent of psychological variables.

Exercise also had a positive effect on wound healing, and this is an indirect measure of systemic inflammation (Emery, Kiecolt-Glaser, Glaser, Malarky, & Frid, 2005). In this study, participants were randomized into exercise and control conditions. They were then brought into the laboratory and given a punch biopsy. The researchers then monitored participants' rate of wound healing. The average number of days for the wound to heal in the exercise group was 29 days. In the control group, it was 38 days. Exercise one hour a day, three days a week lowered perceived stress and improved wound healing. The results of other studies found that wound healing is impaired when stress or hostility levels are high (Kiecolt-Glaser et al., 2005). Stress and hostility both increase systemic inflammation. When systemic inflammation is high, wound healing is impaired because proinflammatory cytokines are in the blood stream and not at the wound site where they belong. The Emery et al. (2005) study indicates that exercise likely improves wound healing by lowering levels of circulating systemic cytokines, thereby increasing them at the wound site.

Overall level of fitness was also related to inflammation in another recent study (Hamer & Steptoe, 2007). The sample was 207 men and women with no history or symptoms of heart disease, and who were not being treated for hypertension, inflammatory disease, or allergy. Participants were given two mentally stressful tasks in the laboratory (a computerized Stroop test or mirror tracing task). Researchers measured heart rate via a submaximal exercise test. A high-systolic blood pressure indicated a low level of fitness. Participants who responded with higher systolic blood pressure to stress also had a higher IL-6 and TNF-α response. The TNF-α response to stress was five times greater in the low-fitness group compared to the high-fitness group. The authors concluded that participants who were physically fit had a lower inflammation response when under stress.

They believed that this was another way that exercise protected individuals from heart disease and other conditions.

A recent study examining the impact of yoga on the inflammatory response also suggests that fitness level did make a difference in the effectiveness of the intervention (Kiecolt-Glaser et al., 2010). In this study, 50 women were exposed to three conditions: yoga, movement control, and passive-video control during three separate visits. There was no overt difference in the inflammatory response following yoga compared to the other exercise types. However, there were large differences based on level of expertise. Yoga novices' level of IL-6 was 41% higher than that of the experts. Likewise, C-reactive protein was 4.75 times higher in yoga novices than that of experts. This difference was likely due to stress the session caused each group. However, the researchers suggested that regular practice could have substantial health benefits.

Psychotherapy

Psychotherapy is another treatment modality for depression that has a long track record of success. In particular, cognitive therapy has been shown to be as effective as medications in treating even major depression. Moreover, patients who received cognitive therapy did better on follow-up, were less likely to relapse, and were less likely to drop out of treatment than those who received medications (Rupke, Blecke, & Renfrow, 2006). Cognitive therapy is based on the premise that distortions in thinking cause depression. It teaches patients to recognize and counter these thoughts (Rupke et al., 2006). The goal is to help patients identify distorted beliefs and replace them with more rational ones.

Anti-Inflammatory Effects of Psychotherapy

Although evidence is quite preliminary, cognitive therapy appears to have an anti-inflammatory effect (Leonard, 2010). Hostility is of interest to the present discussion because it is a particular way of looking at the world. People high in hostility tend to attribute negative motives to others, and have difficulty trusting others and establishing close relationships. It also specifically raises inflammation. As described earlier, hostility was associated with higher levels of IL-1α, IL-1ß, and IL-8 in 44 women, and the combination of depression and hostility led to the highest levels of IL-1ß, IL-8, and TNF-α (Suarez et al., 2004).

Kiecolt-Glaser et al. (2005) found that couples who were high in hostility had higher levels of circulating proinflammatory cytokines. As a result, the rate of wound healing for the high-hostility couples was 60% slower than low-hostility couples. High-hostility couples had fewer cytokines at the wound site, where they were supposed to be, and high levels circulating systemically, where they were more likely to impair health and increase the risk of age-related diseases.

Cognitive therapy specifically addresses beliefs like hostility. Since negative cognitions increase inflammation, we could predict that reducing their occurrence would lower inflammation. That is indeed what Doering and colleagues (2007) found in their study of women after coronary bypass surgery. They found that clinically depressed women had a higher incidence of in-hospital fevers and infections in the six months after surgery, due in part to decreases in Natural Killer cell cytotoxicity. An eight week program of cognitive-behavioral therapy reduced depression, improved Natural Killer cell cytotoxicity, and decreased IL-6 and C-reactive protein. Because the immune system was functioning more effectively, this intervention decreased post-operative infections.

In a study of 45 women newly diagnosed with breast cancer, Thornton et al. (2009) randomly assigned women to either a psychological intervention or control (assessment-only) conditions. The intervention lasted 12 months and the women were assessed at four, eight, and 12 months. Depression and mood state were monitored, as were cell markers of inflammation (white blood cell count, neutrophil count, and helper/suppressor ratio). The results revealed that the psychological intervention significantly reduced pain, depression, fatigue, and inflammation in the women who received it compared to those in the assessment-only condition.

St. John's Wort

Another treatment modality for depression is St. John's wort (*Hypericum perforatum*): the most widely used herbal antidepressant in the world (Dugoua, Mills, Perri, & Koren, 2006). Herbalists have used St. John's wort since the Middle Ages. It derives its name from St. John's Day (June 24) because it blooms near this day on the medieval church calendar. "Wort" is the old English word for a medicinal plant. It is a common wildflower in Great Britain, northern Europe, and northeastern and north central U.S (Balch, 2002).

Mechanism for Efficacy

Researchers still do not understand the exact mechanism for St. John's wort's antidepressant efficacy. St. John's wort is standardized by percentage of hypericin, one of ten active constituents that have been identified so far. Hypericin was once considered the primary antidepressant component, but this is no longer true. Hyperforin is now thought to be the antidepressant constituent (Lawvere & Mahoney, 2005; Muller, 2003; Wurglies & Schubert-Zsilavecz, 2006; Zanoli, 2004). Hyperforin appears to inhibit the reuptake of the serotonin, the same mechanism as the selective serotonin reuptake inhibitors (SSRIs, e.g., fluoxetine, sertraline; Kuhn & Winston, 2000; Werneke, Turner, & Poulton, 2006).

Of interest to our present discussion is that hyperforin is also anti-inflammatory (Dell'Aica, Caniato, Biggin, & Garbisa, 2007; Kuhn & Winston, 2000; Werneke et al., 2006; Wurglies & Schubert-Zsilavecz, 2006). Hyperforin inhibits the expression of intercellular adhesion molecule (Zhou et al., 2004), and it specifically lowers levels of the proinflammatory cytokines involved in depression (Hu et al., 2006). This study used an animal model to test whether St. John's wort could counter the toxic side effects of chemotherapy. The researchers specifically investigated whether St. John's wort had an impact on the levels of proinflammatory cytokines, including IL-1ß, IL-2, IL-6, IFN-γ, and TNF-α. They found that St. John's wort did protect rats receiving chemotherapy by inhibiting proinflammatory cytokines and intestinal epithelium apoptosis. Although not a study of depression, it was the first to demonstrate that St. John's wort inhibits the cytokines that are high in depression.

Antidepressant Medications

The final treatment modality for depression described in this chapter is antidepressants. Until recently, researchers believed that their efficacy was due to their effects on the monoamine neurotransmitters, such as serotonin and norepinephrine (Maes et al., 2009). That conceptualization is accurate, but likely incomplete. Recent studies have noted that antidepressants have some specific anti-inflammatory actions. Moreover, anti-inflammatory drugs appear to have an antidepressant effect and likely modulate the inflammatory response, and this action accounts for their efficacy (Maes et al., 2009; Szelnyi & Vizi, 2007). This suggests that antidepressants have usefulness in the treatment of inflammatory physical diseases, and that anti-inflammatory medications may be useful in depression.

A recent study compared C-reactive protein levels in patients with major depression before and after treatment with selective serotonin reuptake inhibitors (SSRIs). These were cardiac patients taking one of three antidepressant medications following a heart attack: sertraline, fluoxetine, or paroxetine. In these patients, C-reactive protein dropped significantly after treatment, independent of whether depression resolved (O'Brien, Scott, & Dinan, 2006).

An animal model demonstrated the anti-inflammatory and anti-nociceptive (anti-pain) effects of antidepressants in rats. The researchers found that the antidepressant imipramine, amitriptyline, trazadone, and clomipramine were anti-inflammatory as measured by paw edema. Fluoxetine reduced paw edema in a dose-response way. Only sertraline did not reduce edema. In fact, it increased it. The most effective of these medications for pain management were amitriptyline and trazadone (Abdel-Salam, Nofal, & El-Shenawy, 2003).

An in vitro study of inflammation was designed to test whether the antidepressant venlafaxine would modulate the inflammatory response (Vollmar, Haghikia, Dermietzel, & Faustmann, 2007). The researchers hypothesized that the norepinephrine-serotonin system modulated inflammatory diseases, such as depression, given the growing body of evidence that antidepressants have immunoregulatory effects. Venlafaxine is a norepinephrine-serotonin reuptake inhibitor. In astroglia-microglia co-culture, they demonstrated that venlafaxine reduced signs of inflammation by decreasing IL-6 and IL-8. They concluded that venlafaxine was anti-inflammatory. They hypothesized the antidepressant effect of this medication might be due to monoamine-mediated immunomodulation.

Another study tested the anti-inflammatory effects of two antidepressants: fluoxetine and desipramine, in two animal models of human disease: septic shock and allergic asthma (Roumestan et al., 2007). The authors noted that antidepressants affected anti-inflammatory signals and might be useful adjuncts to treatments for these conditions. They also noted that part of antidepressants' efficacy could be due to attenuating brain expression or action of the proinflammatory cytokines. Antidepressants also decrease peripheral inflammation. In their model of septic shock, both antidepressants decreased TNF-α levels. In a model of allergic asthma, they found that fluoxetine and the steroid prednisolone reduced several types of leukocytes, including macrophages, lymphocytes, neutrophils, and eosinophils. Desipramine reduced only macrophages. The authors concluded that antidepressants had a direct peripheral anti-inflammatory effect. They noted that antidepressants can be useful in treating inflammatory conditions—especially those with co-morbid depression, noting that antidepressants may be steroid sparing.

Antidepressants also increase glucocorticoid receptor function and decrease IL-1ß and TNF-α. Some antidepressants that have shown these effects include desipramine, clomipramine, fluoxetine, paroxetine, and citalopram (Pace et al., 2007). Inflammatory cytokines, such as IL-1 and TNF-α, induce the secretion of the prostaglandin COX-2. In contrast, when COX-2 is inhibited, this helps regulate glucocorticoid receptor function as it relates to inflammation and stress-induced neuroendocrine pathways. Anti-inflammatory COX-2 inhibitors (such as Celebrex) enhance glucocorticoid resistance and could explain why COX-2 inhibitors boost the effectiveness of the antidepressant reboxetine in patients with major depression. COX-2 is a signaling molecule that can contribute to glucocorticoid resistance. Pace and colleagues (2007), and more recently Maes and colleagues (2009), recommended that future therapies target these immunologic processes that are relevant to the pathophysiology of psychiatric disorders, such as depression.

Conclusions

Inflammation has become a significant part of an important paradigm shift regarding the etiology of chronic disease. Maes and colleagues (2009) cite depression as a case in point. For many years, researchers assumed that depression was due to serotonin levels and that belief guided the development of medications that influence serotonin levels. Serotonin levels are no doubt involved, but there is likely another underlying mechanism. Maes et al. proposed that it is inflammation. Once inflammation is specifically targeted, the focus of intervention changes, as the studies we have cited in this chapter have demonstrated. That cognitive shift opens up a whole new world of possibilities for preventing and treating chronic diseases and using existing medications in novel ways (such as using antidepressants to treat allergic or inflammatory conditions).

It is within this context that we can appreciate the lifetime health effects of breastfeeding. Breastfeeding can be characterized as something that mothers can do that will improve their health–something that perhaps has similar long-term effects to exercise, Omega-3s, psychotherapy, and treated depression.

Epilogue

As we write this, there has, once again, been a great deal of public debate about whether we are putting "too much pressure" on mothers to breastfeed. Some opponents of breastfeeding state that we need to give mothers who are struggling "permission to wean." The "permission" issue comes up frequently in conversations about postpartum depression. "After all, formula feeding is nearly as good...."

Having heard that argument many times, we have to wonder whether these folks would be so cavalier if they really knew what they were talking about. Obviously, no mother should ever be "forced" to breastfeed. And it is a very sad thing when mothers who want to breastfeed are given no support and are therefore not able to do it. But we also need to recognize–and clearly state–that when women do not breastfeed, they increase their risk of serious, and perhaps lethal, illness as they age. The evidence is overwhelming in support of this point. Even in the short-term, breastfeeding protects both their physical and mental well-being. Breastfeeding is a qualitatively different experience than even mixed feeding, and certainly different than formula feeding. On every measure of well-being, breastfeeding women do better. And thanks to the many researchers in the field of psychoneuroimmunology, we are beginning to understand why this is so.

References

Abdel-Salam, O. M., Nofal, S. M., & El-Shenawy, S. M. (2003). Evaluation of the anti-inflammatory and anti-nociceptive effects of different antidepressants in the rat. *Pharmacology Research, 48*(2), 157-165.

Adcock, I. M., Ito, K., & Barnes, P. J. (2004). Glucocorticoids: Effects on gene transcription. *Proceedings of the American Thoracic Society, 1,* 247-254.

Agren, G., Lundeberg, T., Uvnas-Moberg, K., & Sato, A. (1995). The oxytocin antagonist 1-deamino-2-D-Tyr-(Oet)-4-Thr-8-Orn-oxytocin reverses the increase in the withdrawal response latency to thermal, but not mechanical nociceptive stimuli following oxytocin administration or massage-like stroking in rats. *Neuroscience Letter, 187*(1), 49-52.

Altemus, M., Deuster, P. A., Galliven, E., Carter, C. S., & Gold, P. W. (1995). Suppression of hypothalmic-pituitary-adrenal axis responses to stress in lactating women. *Journal of Clinical Endocrinology and Metabolism, 80*(10), 2954-2959.

Atkinson, H. C., & Waddell, B. J. (1995). The hypothalamic-pituitary-adrenal axis in rat pregnancy and lactation: circadian variation and interrelationship of plasma adrenocorticotropin and corticosterone. *Endocrinology, 136*(2), 512-520.

Babyak, M., Blumenthal, J.A., Herman, S., Khatri, P., Doraiswamy, M., Moore, K., et al. (2000). Exercise treatment for major depression: Maintenance of therapeutic benefit at ten months. *Psychosomatic Medicine, 62,* 633-638.

Balch, P. (2002). *Prescription for herbal healing.* New York: Avery.

Baron, S., Peake, R., James, D., Susman, M., Kennedy, C., Singleton, M., Schuenke, S. (Ed.). (1996). *Medical Microbiology* (4th ed.). The University of Texas Medical Branch at Galveston.

Batten, S. V., Aslan, M., Maciejewski, P. K., & Mazure, C. M. (2004). Childhood maltreatment as a risk factor for adult cardiovascular disease and depression. *Journal of Clinical Psychiatry, 65,* 249-254.

Beutler, B. (2004). Innate immunity: an overview. *Molecular Immunology, 40*(12), 845-859.

Bethin, K. E., Vogt, S. K., & Muglia, L. J. (2000). Interleukin-6 is an essential, corticotropin-releasing hormone--independent stimulator of the adrenal axis during immune system activation. *Proceedings of the National Academy of Sciences USA, 97,* 9317-9322.

Bierhaus, A., Humpert, P., & Nawroth, P. (2006). Linking stress to inflammation. *Anesthesiology Clinics, 24,* 325-340.

Blandino, P., Jr., Barnum, C. J., & Deak, T. (2006). The involvement of norepinephrine and microglia in hypothalamic and splenic IL-1 beta responses to stress. *Journal of Neuroimmunology, 173*, 87-95.

Blumenthal, J. A., Babyak, M.A., Doraiswamy, P.M., Watkins, L., Hoffman, B.M., Barbour, K.A., et al. (2007). Exercise and pharmacotherapy in the treatment of major depressive disorder. *Psychosomatic Medicine, 69*, 587-596.

Bluthe, R. M., Michaud, B., Poli, V., & Dantzer, R. (2000). Role of IL-6 in cytokine-induced sickness behavior: A study with IL-6 deficient mice. *Physiology & Behavior, 70*, 367-373.

Blyton, D. M., Sullivan, C. E., & Edwards, N. (2002). Lactation is associated with an increase in slow-wave sleep in women. *Journal of Sleep Research, 11*(4), 297-303.

Boscarino, J. (1996). Posttraumatic stress disorder, exposure to combat, and lower plasma cortisol among Vietnam veterans: Findings and clinical implications. *Journal of Consulting & Clinical Psychology, 64*, 191-201.

Bosch, O. J. (2011). Maternal nurturing is dependent on her innate anxiety: The behavioral roles of brain oxytocin and vasopressin. *Hormones and Behavior, 59*(2), 202-212.

Brandtzaeg, P. (1998). Development and basic mechanisms of human gut immunity. *Nutrition Reviews, 56*, S5-18.

Brown, S., & Lumley, J. (1998). Maternal health after childbirth: results of an Australian population based survey. *British Journal of Obstetrics and Gynaecology, 105*(2), 156-161.

Brunn, J. M., Lihn, A. S., Verdich, C., Pedersen, S. B., Toubro, S., Astrup, A., et al. (2003). Regulation of adiponecin by adipose tissue-derived cytokines: in vivo and in vitro investigations in humans. *American Journal Physioly Endocrinology Metabolism, 285*, E527-E533.

Bryan, D. L., Hart, P. H., Forsyth, K. D., & Gibson, R. A. (2007). Immunomodulatory constituents of human milk change in response to infant bronchiolitis. *Pediatric Allergy and Immunology, 18*(6), 495-502.

Burger, D., & Dayer, J. M. (2002). Cytokines, acute-phase proteins, and hormones: IL-1 and TNF-α production in contact-mediated activation of monocytes by T lymphocytes. *Annals of the New York Academy of Sciences, 966*, 464-473.

Burnol, A. F., Guerre-Millo, M., Lavau, M., & Girard, J. (1986). Effect of lactation on insulin sensitivity of glucose metabolism in rat adipocytes. *FEBS Letters,194*(2), 292-296.

Byrnes, E. M., Rigero, B. A., & Bridges, R. S. (2000). Opioid receptor antagonism during early lactation results in the increased duration of nursing bouts. *Physilogy and Behavior, 70*(1-2), 211-216.

Callahan, S., Sejourne, N., & Denis, A. (2006). Fatigue and breastfeeding: An inevitable partnership? *Journal of Human Lactation, 22*(2), 182-187.

Cao, Y., Rao, S. D., Phillips, T. M., Umbach, D. M., Bernbaum, J. C., Archer, J. I., et al. (2009). Are breast-fed infants more resilient? Feeding method and cortisol in infants. *Journal of Pediatrics, 154*(3), 452-454.

Cappuccio, F. P., Taggart, F. M., Kandala, N. B., Currie, A., Peile, E., Stranges, S., & Miller, M. A. (2008). Meta-analysis of short sleep duration and obesity in children and adults. *Sleep, 31*(5), 19-26.

Carney, R. M., Freedland, K. E., Steinmeyer, B., Blumenthal, J. A., de Jonge, P., Davidson, K. W., Czajkowski, S. M., et al. (2009). History of depression and survival after acute myocardial infarction. *Psychosomatic Medicine, 71*, 253-259.

Carter, C.S., & Altemus, M. (1997). Integrative functions of lactational hormones in social behavior and stress management. Annals of the New York Acadmeny of Sciences, 15(807), 164-174.

Challis, J. R., Lockwood, C. J., Myatt, L., Norma, J. E., Strauss, J. F., & Petraglia, F. (2009). Inflammation and pregnancy. *Reproductive Sciences, 16*(2), 206-215.

Choquet, M., Darves-Bornoz, J. M., Ledoux, S., Manfredi, R., & Hassler, C. (1997). Self-reported health and behavioral problems among adolescent victims of rape in France: Results of a cross-sectional survey. *Child Abuse and Neglect, 21*, 823-832.

Colson, S. D., Meek, J. H., & Hawdon, J. M. (2008). Optimal positions for the release of primitive neonatal reflexes stimulating breastfeeding. *Early Human Development, 84*(7), 441-449.

Cook, C. J. (1997). Oxytocin and prolactin suppress cortisol responses to acute stress in both lactating and non-lactating sheep. *Journal of Dairy Research, 64*(3), 327-339.

Cook, N., Buring, J., & Ridker, P. (2006). The effect of including C-reactive protein in cardiovascular risk prediction models for women. *Annals of Internal Medicine, 145*, 21-29.

Coussons-Read, M. E., Okun, M.L., Schmitt, M.P., & Giese, S. (2005). Prenatal stress alters cytokine levels in a manner that may endanger human pregnancy. *Psychosomatic Medicine, 67*, 625-631.

Cox, D. B., Kent, J. C., Casey, T. M., Owens, R. A., & Hartmann, P. E. (1999). Breast growth and the urinary excretion of lactose during human pregnancy and early lactation: endocrine relationships. *Experimental Physiology, 84*(2), 421-434.

da Costa, A. P., Wood, S., Ingram, C. D., & Lightman, S. L. (1996). Region-specific reduction in stress-induced c-fos mRNA expression during pregnancy and lactation. *Brain Research, 742*(1-2), 177-184.

Danese, A., Moffitt, T. E., Harrington, H., Milne, B. J., Polanczyk, G., Pariante, C. M., & Caspi, A. (2009). Adverse childhood experiences and adult risk factors for age-related disease: Depression, inflammation, and clustering of metabolic risk factors. *Archives of Pediatric & Adolescent Medicine, 163*(12), 1135-1143.

Danese, A., Pariante, C. M., Caspi, A., Taylor, A., & Poulton, R. (2007). Childhood maltreatment predicts adult inflammation in a life-course study. *Proceedings of the National Academy of Sciences U S A, 104*(4), 1319-1324.

Dantzer, R., & Kelley, K. W. (2007). Twenty years of research on cytokine-induced sickness behavior. *Brain, Behavior & Immunity, 21*, 153-160.

Dayan, J., Creveuil, C., Marks, M.N., Conroy, S., Herlicoviez, M., Dreyfus, M., & Tordjman, S. (2006). Prenatal depression, prenatal anxiety, and spontaneous preterm birth: A prospective cohort study among women with early and regular care. *Psychosomatic Medicine, 68*, 938-946.

de la Rosa, G., Yang, D., Tewary, P., Varadhachary, A., & Oppenheim, J. J. (2008). Lactoferrin acts as an alarmin to promote the recruitment and activation of APCs and antigen-specific immune responses. *Journal of Immunology, 180*(10), 6868-6876.

Dell'Aica, I., Caniato, R., Biggin, S., & Garbisa, S. (2007). Matrix proteases, green tea, and St. John's wort: Biomedical research catches up with folk medicine. *Clinical Chimica Acta, 381*, 69-77.

Dennis, C. L., & McQueen, K. (2009). The relationship between infant-feeding outcomes and postpartum depression: A qualitative systematic review. *Pediatrics, 123*, e736-e751.

Derzsy, Z., Prohaszka, Z., Rigo, J., Fust, G., & Molvarec, A. (2010). Activation of the complement system in normal pregnancy and preeclampsia. *Molecular Immunity, 47*(7-8), 1500-1506.

Deschamps, S., Woodside, B., & Walker, C. D. (2003). Pups presence eliminates the stress hyporesponsiveness of early lactating females to a psychological stress representing a threat to the pups. *Journal of Neuroendocrinology, 15*(5), 486-497.

Detillion, C., Hunzeker, J., Craft, T., Tseng, R., Sheridan, J., DeVries, C (2003). Wound healing is affected by parturition and lactation [Abstract]. *Society for Neuroscience Annual meeting.* New Orleans, LA.

Detillion, C. E., Craft, T. K., Glasper, E. R., Prendergast, B. J., & DeVries, A. C. (2004). Social facilitation of wound healing. *Psychoneuroendocrinology, 29*(8), 1004-1011.

Dewey, K. G., Nommsen-Rivers, L. A., Heinig, M. J., & Cohen, R. J. (2003). Risk factors for suboptimal infant breastfeeding behavior, delayed onset of lactation, and excess neonatal weight loss. *Pediatrics, 112*(3 Pt 1), 607-619.

Dhabhar, F. D., & McEwen, B.S. (2001). Bidirectional effects of stress and glucocorticoid hormones on immune function: Possible explanations for paradoxical observations. In R. Ader, D.L. Felten, & N. Cohen (Eds.), *Psychoneuroimmunology: Vol. 1* (3rd ed., pp. 301-338). New York: Academic Press.

Doan, T., Gardiner, A., Gay, C. L., & Lee, K. A. (2007). Breastfeeding increases sleep duration of new parents. *Journal of Perinatal & Neonatal Nursing, 21*(3), 200-206.

Dobie, D. J., Maynard, C., Kivlahan, D. R., Johnson, K. M., Simpson, T., David, A. C., & Bradley, K. (2006). Posttraumatic stress disorder screening status is associated with increased VA medical and surgical utilization in women. *Journal of General Internal Medicine, 21 Suppl 3*, S58-64.

Doering, L. V., Cross, R., Vredevoe, D., Martinez-Maza, O.l., & Cowan, M.J. (2007). Infection, depression and immunity in women after coronary artery bypass: A pilot study of cognitive behavioral therapy. *Alternative Therapy, Health & Medicine, 13*, 18-21.

Dorheim, S. K., Bondevik, G. T., Eberhard-Gran, M., & Bjorvatn, B. (2009). Sleep and depression in postpartum women: A population-based study. *Sleep, 32*(7), 847-855.

Dugoua, J. J., Mills, E., Perri, D., & Koren, G. (2006). Safety and efficacy of St. John's wort (Hypericum) during pregnancy and lactation. *Canadian Journal of Clinical Pharmacology, 13*, e268-e276.

Elenkov, I. J., Hoffman, J., & Wilder, R. L. (1997). Does differential neuroendocrine control of cytokine production govern the expression of autoimmune diseases in pregnancy and the postpartum period? *Molecular Medicine Today, 3*(9), 379-383.

Elovainio, M., Pulkki-Raback, L., Kivimaki, M., Jokela, M., Viikari, J. S., Raitakari, O. T., & Telama, R. (2010). Lipid trajectories as predictors of depressive symptoms: The Young Finns study. *Health Psychology, 29*(3), 237-245.

Emery, C. F., Kiecolt-Glaser, J.K., Glaser, R., Malarky, W.B., & Frid, D.J. (2005). Exercise accelerates wound healing among health older adults: A preliminary investigation. *The Journals of Gerontology: Medical Sciences, 60A*, 1432-1436.

Erbagci, A. B., Cekmen, M. B., Balat, O., Balat, A., Aksoy, F., & Tarakcioglu, M. (2005). Persistency of high proinflammatory cytokine levels from colostrum to mature milk in preeclampsia. *Clinical Biochemistry, 38*(8), 712-716.

Everson-Rose, S. A., Lewis, T. T., Karavolos, K., Dugan, S. A., Wesley, D., & Powell, L. H. (2009). Depressive symptoms and increased visceral fat in middle-aged women. *Psychosomatic Medicine, 71*, 410-416.

Felitti, V. J., Anda, R. F., Nordenberg, D., Williamson, D. F., Spitz, A. M., Edwards, V., et al. (2001). Relationship of childhood abuse and household dysfunction to many of the leading causes of death in adults. In K. Franey, R. Geffner & R. Falconer (Eds.), *The cost of child maltreatment: Who pays? We all do* (pp. 53-69). San Diego, CA: Family Violence and Sexual Assault Institute.

Ferrucci, L., Cherubini, A., Bandinelli, S., Bartali, B., Corsi A., Lauretani, F., et al. (2006). Relationship of plasma polyunsaturated fatty acids to circulating inflammatory markers. *Journal of Clinical Endocrinology & Metabolism, 91*, 439-446.

Field, T., & Diego, M. (2008). Cortisol: The culprit prenatal stress variable. *International Journal of Neuroscience, 118*(8), 1181-1205.

Field, T., Diego, M., Hernandez-Reif, M., Figueiredo, B., Ezell, S., & Siblalingappa, V. (2010). Depressed mothers and infants are more relaxed during breastfeeding versus bottlefeeding interactions: brief report. *Infant Behavior and Development, 33*(2), 241-244.

Fischer, D., Patchev, V. K., Hellbach, S., Hassan, A. H., & Almeida, O. F. (1995). Lactation as a model for naturally reversible hypercorticalism plasticity in the mechanisms governing hypothalamo-pituitary- adrenocortical activity in rats. *Journal of Clinical Investigation, 96*(3), 1208-1215.

Franceschini, R., Venturini, P. L., Cataldi, A., Barreca, T., Ragni, N., & Rolandi, E. (1989). Plasma beta-endorphin concentrations during suckling in lactating women. *British Journal of Obstetrics and Gynaecology, 96*(6), 711-713.

Frasure-Smith, N., & Lesperance, F. (2005). Reflections on depression as a cardiac risk factor. *Psychosomatic Medicine, 67*, S19-S25.

Freeman, M. P., Hibbeln, J.R., Wisner, K.L., Davis, J.M., Mischoulon, D., Peet, M., et al. (2006). Omega-3 fatty acids: Evidence basis for treatment and future research in psychiatry. *Journal of Clinical Psychiatry, 67*, 1954-1967.

Gallo, L. C., Troxel, W.M., Matthews, K.A., & Kuller, L.H. (2003). Marital status and quality in middle-aged women: Associations with levels and trajectories of cardiovascular risk factors. *Health Psychology, 22*, 453-463.

Gay, C. L., Lee, K. A., & Lee, S. Y. (2004). Sleep patterns and fatigue in new mothers and fathers. *Biological Research for Nursing, 5*(4), 311-318.

Giles, T. (2005). Relevance of blood pressure variation in the circadian onset of cardiovascular events. *Journal of Hypertension, 23 (Suppl.1)*, S35-S39.

Gjerdingen, D. K., & Center, B. A. (2003). First-time parents' prenatal to postpartum changes in health, and the relation of postpartum health to work and partner characteristics. *Journal of the American Board of Family Practitioners, 16*(4), 304-311.

Goebel, M. U., Mills, P.J., Irwin, M.R., & Ziegler, M.G. (2000). Interleukin-6 and tumor necrosis factor-alpha production after acute psychological stress, exercise, and infused isoproterenol: Differential effects and pathways. *Psychosomatic Research, 62*, 591-598.

Goedhart, G., Snijders, A. C., Hesselink, A. E., van Poppel, M. N., Bonsel, G. J., & Vridkotte, T. G. M. (2010). Maternal depressive symptoms in relation to perinatal mortality and morbidity: Results from a large multiethnic cohort study. *Psychosomatic Medicine, 72*, 769-776.

Gold, P., Goodman, F., & Chrousos, G. P. (1988). Clinical and biochemical manifestations of depression: Relation to the neurobiology of stress (1). *The New England Journal of Medicine, 319*, 348-353.

Goldbacher, E. M., Bromberger, J., & Matthews, K. A. (2009). Lifetime history of major depression predicts the development of the metabolic syndrome in middle-aged women. *Psychosomatic Medicine, 71*, 266-272.

Goyal, D., Gay, C. L., & Lee, K. A. (2009). Fragmented maternal sleepis more strongly correlated wtih depressive symptoms than infant temperament at three months postpartum. *Archives of Women's Mental Health, 12*, 229-237.

Gregory, R. L., Wallace, J. P., Gfell, L. E., Marks, J., & King, B. A. (1997). Effect of exercise on milk immunoglobulin A. *Medicine and Science in Sports and Exercise,29*(12), 1596-1601.

Groer, M. W., Davis, M. W., & Hemphill, J. (2002). Postpartum stress: Current concepts and the possible protective role of breastfeeding. *Journal of Obstetric, Gynecologic, & Neonatal Nursing, 31*(4), 411-417.

Groer, M., Davis, M., & Steele, K. (2004). Associations between human milk SIgA and maternal immune, infectious, endocrine, and stress variables. *Journal of Human Lactation, 20*(2), 153-158; quiz 159-163.

Groer, M., El-Badri, N., Djeu, J., Harrington, M., & Van Eepoel, J. (2009). Suppression of natural killer cell cytotoxicity in postpartum women. *American Journal of Reproductive Immunology, 63*(3), 209-213.

Groer, M. W. (2005). Differences between exclusive breastfeeders, formula-feeders, and controls: a study of stress, mood, and endocrine variables. *Biological Research for Nursing, 7*(2), 106-117.

Groer, M. W., Beckstead, J. W. (2011). Multidimensional scaling of Human Milk Cytokines. *Biological Research for Nursing,* in press.

Groer, M. W., Davis, M. W., Smith, K., Casey, K., Kramer, V., & Bukovsky, E. (2005). Immunity, inflammation and infection in post-partum breast and formula feeders. *American Journal of Reproductive Immunology, 54*(4), 222-231.

Groer, M. W., Manion, M., Szekeres, C., & El-Badri, N. S. (2011). Fetal Microchimerism and Women's Health: A new paradigm. *Biological Research for Nursing,* in press.

Groer, M. W., & Morgan, K. (2007). Immune, health and endocrine characteristics of depressed postpartum mothers. *Psychoneuroendocrinology, 32*(2), 133-139.

Groer, M. W., & Shelton, M. M. (2009). Exercise is associated with elevated proinflammatory cytokines in human milk. *Journal of Obstetrics, Gynecology and Neonatal Nursing, 38*(1), 35-41.

Groer, M. W., Thomas, S. P., Evans, G. W., Helton, S., & Weldon, A. (2006). Inflammatory effects and immune system correlates of rape. *Violence and Victims, 21*(6), 796-808.

Groer, M.W. (2011). [Inflammatory response at birth.] Unpublished raw data.

Grundy, S. M., Cleeman, J. I., Merz, C. N., Brewer, H. B., Jr., Clark, L. T., Hunninghake, D. B., et al. (2004). Implications of recent clinical trials for the National Cholesterol Education Program Adult Treatment Panel III Guidelines. *Journal of the American College of Cardiology, 44*(3), 720-732.

Gunderson, E. P., Jacobs, D. R., Chiang, V., Lewis, C. E., Feng, J., Quesenberry, C. P., & Sidney, S. (2010). Duration of lactation and incidence of the metabolic syndrome in women of reproductive age according to gestational diabetes mellitus status: A 20-year prospective study in CARDIA (Coronary Artery Risk Development in Young Adults). *Diabetes, 59*(2), 495-504.

Gunnar, M., & Quevedo, K. (2007). The neurobiology of stress and development. *Annual Review of Psychology, 58*, 145-173.

Gutkowska, J., Jankowski, M., Mukaddam-Daher, S., & McCann, S. M. (2000). Corticotropin-releasing hormone causes antidiuresis and antinatriuresis by stimulating vasopressin and inhibiting atrial natriuretic peptide release in male rats. *Proceedings of the National Academy of Sciences U S A,97*(1), 483-488.

Haas, J. S., Jackson, R. A., Fuentes-Afflick, E., Stewart, A. L., Dean, M. L., Brawarsky, P., et al. (2005). Changes in the health status of women during and after pregnancy. *Journal of General Internal Medicine, 20*(1), 45-51.

Hadji, P., Ziller, V., Kalder, M., Gottschalk, M., Hellmeyer, L., Hars, O., et al. (2002). Influence of pregnancy and breast-feeding on quantitative ultrasonometry of bone in postmenopausal women. *Climacteric, 5*(3), 277-285.

Haffner, S., & Taegtmeyer, H. (2003). Epidemic obesity and the metabolic syndrome. *Circulation, 108*, 1541-1545.

Hall, I. J., Moorman, P. G., Millikan, R. C., & Newman, B. (2005). Comparative analysis of breast cancer risk factors among African-American women and White women. *American Journal of Epidemiology, 161*(1), 40-51.

Hall, M. H., Muldoon, M. F., Jennings, J. R., Buysse, D. J., Flory, J. D., & Manuck, S. B. (2008). Self-reported sleep duration is associated with the metabolic syndrome in midlife adults. *Sleep, 31*(5), 635-643.

Halonen, M., Lohman, I. C., Stern, D. A., Spangenberg, A., Anderson, D., Mobley, S., et al. (2009). Th1/Th2 patterns and balance in cytokine production in the parents and infants of a large birth cohort. *Journal of Immunology,182*(5), 3285-3293.

Hamazaki, K., Itomura, M., Huan, M., Nishizawa, H., Sawazaki, S., Tanouchi, M., et al. (2005). Effect of omega-3 fatty acid-containing phospholipids on blood catecholamine concentrations in healthy volunteers: A randomized, placebo-controlled, double-blind trial. *Nutrition, 21*, 705-710.

Hamer, M., & Steptoe, A. (2007). Association between physical fitness, parasympathetic control, and proinflammatory responses to mental stress. *Psychosomatic Medicine, 69*, 660-666.

Handlin, L., Jonas, W., Petersson, M., Ejdeback, M., Ransjo-Arvidson, A. B., Nissen, E., et al. (2009). Effects of sucking and skin-to-skin contact on maternal ACTH and cortisol levels during the second day postpartum-influence of epidural analgesia and oxytocin in the perinatal period. *Breastfeeding Medicine, 4*(4), 207-220.

Hanson, L. A., & Korotkova, M. (2002). The role of breastfeeding in prevention of neonatal infection. *Seminars in Neonatology, 7*(4), 275-281.

Haram, K., Augensen, K., & Elsayed, S. (1983). Serum protein pattern in normal pregnancy with special reference to acute-phase reactants. *British Journal of Obstetrics and Gynaecology, 90*, 139-145.

Harris, B., Lovett, L., Smith, J., Read, G., Walker, R., & Newcombe, R. (1996). Cardiff puerperal mood and hormone study. III. Postnatal depression at 5 to 6 weeks postpartum, and its hormonal correlates across the peripartum period. *British Journal of Psychiatry, 168*(6), 739-744.

Heinrichs, M., Meinlschmidt, G., Neumann, I., Wagner, S., Kirschbaum, C., Ehlert, U., & Hellhammer, D. H. (2001). Effects of suckling on hypothalamic-pituitary-adrenal axis responses to psychosocial stress in postpartum lactating women. *Journal of Clinical Endocrinology & Metabolism, 86*, 4798-4804.

Higuchi, T., Negoro, H., & Arita, J. (1989). Reduced responses of prolactin and catecholamine to stress in the lactating rat. *Journal of Endocrinology,122*(2), 495-498.

Howren, M. B., Lamkin, D. M., & Suls, J. (2009). Associations of depression with C-reactive protein, IL-1, and IL-6: A meta-analysis. *Psychosomatic Medicine, 71*, 171-186.

Hu, Z. P., Yang, X.X., Chan, S.Y., Xu A.L., Duan, W., Zhu, Y.Z., et al. (2006). St. John's wort attenuates irinotecan-induced diarrhea via down-regulation of intestinal pro-inflammatory cytokines and inhibition of intestinal epithelial apoptosis. *Toxicology & Applied Pharmacology, 216*, 225-237.

Huang, Q. H., Takaki, A., & Arimura, A. (1997). Central noradrenergic system modulates plasma interleukin-6 production by peripheral interleukin-1. *American Journal of Physiology--Regulatory, Integrative, and Comparative Physiology, 273*, R731-R738.

Hulme, P. A. (2000). Symptomatology and health care utilization of women primary care patients who experienced childhood sexual abuse. *Child Abuse and Neglect, 24*, 1471-1484.

Humphreys, J. C., Lee, K. A., Neylan, T. C., & Marmar, C. R. (1999). Sleep patterns of sheltered battered women. *Journal of Nursing Scholarship, 31*, 139-143.

Ip, S., Chung, M., Raman, G., Chew, P., Magula, N., DeVine, D., et al. (2007). Breastfeeding and maternal and infant health outcomes in developed countries. *Evidence Report/Technology Assessment (Full Report), 153*, 1-186.

Israel, E. J. (1994). Neonatal necrotizing enterocolitis, a disease of the immature intestinal mucosal barrier. *Acta Paediatrica Suppl, 396*, 27-32.

Jaedicke, K. M., Fuhrmann, M. D., & Stefanski, V. (2009). Lactation modifies stress-induced immune changes in laboratory rats. *Brain Behavior and Immunity, 23*(5), 700-708.

Jensen, R. G. (Ed.). (1995). *Handbook of milk composition.* San Diego, CA.

Jevitt, C., Hernandez, I., & Groer, M. (2007). Lactation complicated by overweight and obesity: Supporting the mother and newborn. *Journal of Midwifery and Womens Health, 52*(6), 606-613.

Johnson, J. D., Campisi, J., Sharkey, C. M., Kennedy, S. L., Nickerson, M., Greenwood, B. N., & Flesner, M. (2005). Catecholamines mediate stress-induced increases in peripheral and central inflammatory cytokines. *Neuroscience, 135*, 1295-1307.

Kaneita, Y., Uchiyama, M., Yoshiike, N., & Ohida, T. (2008). Associations of usual sleep duration with serum lipid and lipoprotein levels. *Sleep, 31*(5), 645-652.

Kendall-Tackett, K. A. (2003). *Treating the lifetime health effects of childhood victimization.* Kingston, NJ: Civic Research Institute.

Kendall-Tackett, K. A. (2007a). A new paradigm for depression in new mothers: The central role of inflammation and how breastfeeding and anti-inflammatory treatments protect maternal mental health. *International Breastfeeding Journal, 2:6*(http://www.internationalbreastfeedingjournal.com/content/2/1/6).

Kendall-Tackett, K. A. (2007b). Cardiovascular disease and metabolic syndrome as sequelae of violence against women: A psychoneuroimmunology approach. *Trauma, Violence and Abuse, 8*, 117-126.

Kendall-Tackett, K. A. (2009). Psychological trauma and physical health: A psychoneuroimmunology approach to etiology of negative heatlh effects and possible interventions. *Psychological Trauma, 1*(1), 35-48.

Kendall-Tackett, K. A. (2010a). *Depression in new mothers: Causes, consequences and treatment options, 2nd Edition.* London: Routledge.

Kendall-Tackett, K. A. (2010b). Long-chain omega-3 fatty acids and women's mental health in the perinatal period. *Journal of Midwifery and Women's Health, 55*(6), 561-567.

Kendall-Tackett, K. A. (2011). Do recent research findings mean that mothers should not take Omega-3s? *Clinical Lactation, 2*(1), 34-36.

Kendall-Tackett, K.A., Cong, Z., & Hale, T.W. (2011). Breastfeeding lowers maternal fatigue or depression risk. *Clinical Lactation, 2*(2). 22-26.

Kiecolt-Glaser, J. K., Belury, M.A., Porter, K., Beversdoft, D., Lemeshow, S., & Glaser, R. (2007). Depressive symptoms, omega-6: omega-3 fatty acids, and inflammation in older adults. *Psychosomatic Medicine, 69*, 217-224.

Kiecolt-Glaser, J. K., Christian, L., Preston, H., Houts, C., Malarkey, W. B., Emery, C. F., & Glaser, R. (2010). Stress, inflammation, and yoga practice. *Psychosomatic Medicine, 72*(2), 113-121.

Kiecolt-Glaser, J. K., Loving, T.J., Stowell, J.R., Malarky, W.B., Lemeshow, S., Dickinson, S.L., & Glaser, R. (2005). Hostile marital interactions, proinflammatory cytokine production, and wound healing. *Archives of General Psychiatry, 62*, 1377-1384.

Kiecolt-Glaser, J. K., & Newton, T. L. (2001). Marriage and health: His and hers. *Psychological Bulletin, 127*, 472-503.

Kip, K. E., Marroquin, O. C., Kelley, D. E., Johnson, B. D., Kelsey, S. F., Shaw, L. J., et al. (2004). Clinical importance of obesity versus the metabolic syndrome in cardiovascular risk in women: A report from the Women's Ischemia Syndrome Evaluation (WISE) study. *Circulation, 109*(6), 706-713.

Kliegman, R. M., Walker, W. A., & Yolken, R. H. (1993). Necrotizing enterocolitis: Research agenda for a disease of unknown etiology and pathogenesis. *Pediatric Research, 34*(6), 701-708.

Kohut, M. L., McCann, D.A., Konopka, D.W.R., Cunnick, J.E., Franke, W.D., Castillo, M.C., & Vanderah, R.E. (2006). Aerobic exercise, but not flexibility/resistance exercise, reduces serum IL-18, CRP, and IL-6 independent of ß-blockers, BMI, and psychosocial factors in older adults. *Brain, Behavior, & Immunity, 20*, 201-209.

Kop, W. J., Gottdiener, J. S., Tangen, C. M., Fried, L. P., McBurnie, M. A., Walston, J., et al. (2002). Inflammation and coagulation factors in persons > 65 years of age with symptoms of depression but without evidence of myocardial ischemia. *American Journal of Cardiology, 89*(4), 419-424.

Kozak, W., Kluger, M. J., Tesfaigzi, J., Kozak, A., Mayfield, K. P., Wachulec, M., et al. (2000). Molecular mechanisms of fever and endogenous antipyresis. *Annals of the New York Academy of Sciences, 917*, 121-134.

Krakow, B., Artar, A., Warner, T. D., Melendrez, D., Johnston, L., Hollifield, M., et al. (2000a). Sleep disorder, depression, and suicidality in female sexual assault survivors. *Crisis, 21*(4), 163-170.

Krakow, B., Lowry, C., Germain, A., Gaddy, L., Hollifield, M., Koss, M., et al. (2000b). A retrospective study on improvements in nightmares and post-traumatic stress disorder following treatment for co-morbid sleep-disordered breathing. *Journal of Psychosomatic Research, 49*(5), 291-298.

Kroenke, K., & Mangelsdorff, A. D. (1989). Common symptoms in ambulatory care: incidence, evaluation, therapy, and outcome. *American Journal of Medicine, 86*(3), 262-266.

Kubzansky, L. D., Davidson, K. W., & Rozanski, A. (2005). The clinical impact of negative psychological states: expanding the spectrum of risk for coronary artery disease. *Psychosomatic Medicine, 67 Suppl 1*, S10-14.

Kuhn, M. A., & Winston, D. (2000). *Herbal therapy and supplements: A scientific and traditional approach*. Philadelphia, PA: Lippincott.

Lakka, T. A., Lakka, H. M., Rankinen, T., Leon, A. S., Rao, D. C., Skinner, J. S., et al. (2005). Effect of exercise training on plasma levels of C-reactive protein in healthy adults: the HERITAGE Family Study. *European Heart Journal, 26*(19), 2018-2025.

Landys, M., Ramenofsky, M., & Wingfield, J. C. (2006). Actions of glucocorticoids at a seasonal baseline as compared to stress-related levels in the regulation of periodic life processes. *General and Comparative Endocrinology, 148*, 132-149.

Lankarani-Fard, A., Kritz-Silverstein, D., Barrett-Connor, E., & Goodman-Gruen, D. (2001). Cumulative duration of breast-feeding influences cortisol levels in postmenopausal women. *Journal of Womens Health and Gender Based Medicine, 10*(7), 681-687.

Lawvere, S., & Mahoney, M.C. (2005). St. John's wort. *American Family Physician, 72*, 2249-2254.

LeMay, L. G., Otterness, I. G., Vander, A. J., & Kluger, M. J. (1990). In vivo evidence that the rise in plasma IL-6 following injection of a fever-inducing dose of LPS is mediated by IL-1 beta. *Cytokine, 2*, 199-204.

LeMay, L. G., Vander, A. J., & Kluger, M. J. (1990). The effects of psychological stress on plasma interleukin-6 activity in rats. *Physiology & Behavior, 47*, 957-961.

Leonard, B. E. (2010). The concept of depression as a dysfunction of the immune system. *Current Immunology Review, 6*(3), 205-212.

Li, J., Vestergaard, M., Obel, C., Precht, D. H., Christensen, J., Lu, M., & Olsen, J. (2009). Prenatal stress and cerebral palsy: A nationwide cohort study in Denmark. *Psychosomatic Medicine, 71*, 615-618.

Light, K. C., Smith, T. E., Johns, J. M., Brownley, K. A., Hofheimer, J. A., & Amico, J. A. (2000). Oxytocin responsivity in mothers of infants: a preliminary study of relationships with blood pressure during laboratory stress and normal ambulatory activity. *Health Psychology, 19*(6), 560-567.

Lightman, S. L., & Young, W. S., 3rd (1989). Lactation inhibits stress-mediated secretion of corticosterone and oxytocin and hypothalamic accumulation of corticotropin-releasing factor and enkephalin messenger ribonucleic acids. *Endocrinology, 124*(5), 2358-2364.

Lin, E. H. B., Heckbert, S. R., Rutter, C. M., Katon, W. J., Ciechanowski, P., Ludman, E. J., et al. (2009). Depression and increased mortality in diabetes: Unexpected causes of death. *Annals of Family Medicine, 7*(5), 414-421.

Lipworth, L., Bailey, L. R., & Trichopoulos, D. (2000). History of breast-feeding in relation to breast cancer risk: A review of the epidemiologic literature. *Journal of the National Cancer Institute,92*(4), 302-312.

Lund, I., Lundeberg, T., Kurosawa, M., & Uvnas-Moberg, K. (1999). Sensory stimulation (massage) reduces blood pressure in unanaesthetized rats. *Journal of the Autonomic Nervous System, 78*(1), 30-37.

Ma, H., Bernstein, L., Ross, R. K., & Ursin, G. (2006). Hormone-related risk factors for breast cancer in women under age 50 years by estrogen and progesterone receptor status: results from a case-control and a case-case comparison. *Breast Cancer Research, 8*(4), R39.

Maes, M. (2001). Psychological stress and the inflammatory response system. *Clinical Science, 101*, 193-194.

Maes, M., Christophe, A., Bosmans, E., Lin, A., & Neels, H. (2000). In humans, serum polyunsaturated fatty acid levels predict the response of proinflammatory cytokines to psychologic stress. *Biological Psychiatry, 47*, 910-920.

Maes, M., & Smith, R.S. (1998). Fatty acids, cytokines, and major depression. *Biological Psychiatry, 43*, 313-314.

Maes, M., Yirmyia, R., Noraberg, J., Brene, S., Hibblen, J., Perini, G., et al. (2009). The inflammatory & neurodegenerative (I&ND) hypothesis of depression: Leads for future research and new drug development. *Metabolic Brain Disease, 24*, 27-53.

Maestripieri, D., Hoffman, C. L., Fulks, R., & Gerald, M. S. (2008). Plasma cortisol responses to stress in lactating and nonlactating female rhesus macaques. *Hormones and Behavior, 53*(1), 170-176.

Magiakou, M. A., Mastorakos, G., Webster, E., & Chrousos, G. P. (1997). The hypothalamic-pituitary-adrenal axis and the female reproductive system. *Annals of the New York Academy of Sciences, 816*, 42-56.

Maier, S. F., & Watkins, L. R. (1998). Cytokines for psychologists: Bidirectional immune-to-brain communication for understanding behavior, mood, and cognition. *Psychological Review, 105*, 83-107.

Mastorakos, G., & Ilias, I. (2003). Maternal and fetal hypothalamic-pituitary-adrenal axes during pregnancy and postpartum. *Annals of the New York Academy of Sciences, 997*, 136-149.

Matthews, K. A., Schott, L. L., Bromberger, J., Cyranowski, J., Everson-Rose, S. A., & Sowers, M. F. (2007). Associations between depressive symptoms and inflammatory/hemostatic markers in women during the menopausal transition. *Psychosomatic Medicine, 69*(2), 124-130.

Matzinger, P. (2002). The danger model: a renewed sense of self. *Science, 296*(5566), 301-305.

McAuley, E., Blissmer, B., Katula, J., Duncan, T.E., & Mihalko, S.L. (2000). Physical activity, self-esteem, and self-efficacy relationships in older adults: A randomized controlled trial. *Annals of Behavioral Medicine, 22*, 131-139.

McBeth, J., Chiu, Y. H., Silman, A., Ray, D., Morriss, R., Dickens, C., et al. (2005). Hypothalamic-pituitary-adrenal stress axis function and the relationship with chronic widespread pain and its antecedents. *Arthritis Research and Therapeutics, 7*, R992-R1000.

McCarthy, M. M. (1990). Oxytocin inhibits infanticide in female house mice (Mus domesticus). *Hormones and Behavior, 24*(3), 365-375.

McCarthy, M. M., Curran, G. H., & Siegel, H. I. (1994). Evidence for the involvement of prolactin in the maternal behavior of the hamster. *Physiology and Behavior, 55*(1), 181 184.

McEwen, B. S. (2003). Mood disorders and allostatic load. *Biological Psychiatry, 54*, 200-207.

Meinlschmidt, G., Martin, C., Neumann, I. D., & Heinrichs, M. (2010). Maternal cortisol in late pregnancy and hypothalamic-pituitary-adrenal reactivity to psychosocial stress postpartum in women. *Stress, 13*(2), 163-171.

Mezzacappa, E. S., & Katkin, E. S. (2002). Breastfeeding is associated with reduced perceived stress and negative mood in mothers. *Health Psychology, 21*, 187-193.

Mezzacappa, E. S., Kelsey, R. M., Myers, M. M., & Katkin, E. S. (2001). Breast-feeding and maternal cardiovascular function. *Psychophysiology, 38*(6), 988-997.

Mischoulon, D. (2009). Update and critique of natural remedies as antidepressant treatments. *Obstetric & Gynecology Clinics of North America, 36*, 787-807.

Miyake, A., Tahara, M., Koike, K., & Tanizawa, O. (1989). Decrease in neonatal suckled milk volume in diabetic women. *European Journal of Obstetrics, Gynecology and Reproductive Biology, 33*(1), 49-53.

Moorman, A. J., Mozaffarian, D., Wilkinson, C. W., Lawler, R. L., McDonald, G. B., Crane, B. A., et al. (2007). In patients with heart failure elevated soluble TNF-receptor 1 is associated with higher risk of depression. *Journal of Cardiac Failure, 13*(9), 738-743. 10.1016/j.cardfail.2007.06.301

Moos, R. H., & Solomon, G. F. (1964). Personality correlates of the rapidity of progression of rheumatoid arthritis. *Annals of Rheumatic Diseases, 23*, 145-151.

Mor, G., & Cardenas, I. (2010). The immune system in pregnancy: A unique complexity. *American Journal of Reproductive Immunology, 63*(6), 425-433.

Mora, S., Lee, I. M., Buring, J. E., & Ridker, P. M. (2006). Association of physical activity and body mass index with novel and traditional cardiovascular biomarkers in women. *Journal of the American Medical Association, 295*(12), 1412-1419.

Morgans, D. (1995). Bromocriptine and postpartum lactation suppression. *British Journal of Obstetrics and Gynaecology, 102*(11), 851-853.

Morin, C. M., & Ware, J. C. (1996). Sleep and psychopathology. *Applied and Preventive Psychology, 5*, 211-224.

Morrison, B., Ludington-Hoe, S., & Anderson, G. C. (2006). Interruptions to breastfeeding dyads on postpartum day 1 in a university hospital. *Journal of Obsterics, Gynecology and Neonatal Nursing, 35*(6), 709-716.

Muller, W. E. (2003). Current St. John's wort research from mode of action to clinical efficacy. *Pharmacology Research, 47*, 101-109.

Neumann, I. D., Johnstone, H. A., Hatzinger, M., Liebsch, G., Shipston, M., Russell, J. A., et al. (1998). Attenuated neuroendocrine responses to emotional and physical stressors in pregnant rats involve adenohypophysial changes. *Journal of Physiology, 508 (Pt 1)*, 289-300.

Neumann, I. D., Torner, L., & Wigger, A. (2000). Brain oxytocin: differential inhibition of neuroendocrine stress responses and anxiety-related behaviour in virgin, pregnant and lactating rats. *Neuroscience, 95*(2), 567-575.

Neville, M. C., & Morton, J. (2001). Physiology and endocrine changes underlying human lactogenesis II. *Journal of Nutrition, 131*(11), 3005S-3008S.

Newburg, D. S., & Walker, W. A. (2007). Protection of the neonate by the innate immune system of developing gut and of human milk. *Pediatric Research, 61*(1), 2-8.

Nguyen, D. A., & Neville, M. C. (1998). Tight junction regulation in the mammary gland. *Journal of Mammary Gland Biology and Neoplasia, 3*(3), 233-246.

Niaura, R., Banks, S. M., Ward, K. D., Stoney, C. M., Spiro, A., 3rd, Aldwin, C. M., et al. (2000). Hostility and the metabolic syndrome in older males: the normative aging study. *Psychosomatic Medicine, 62*(1), 7-16.

Nissen, E., Lilja, G., Widstrom, A. M., & Uvnas-Moberg, K. (1995). Elevation of oxytocin levels early post partum in women. *Acta Obstetricia et Gynecologica Scandanavica, 74*(7), 530-533.

O'Brien, S. M., Scott, L. V., & Dinan, T. G. (2006). Antidepressant therapy and C-reactive protein levels. *British Journal of Psychiatry, 188*, 449-452.

Oddy, W. H., Kendall, G. E., Li, J., Jacoby, P., Robinson, M., de Klerk, N. H., et al. (2009). The long-term effects of breastfeeding on child and adolescent mental health: A pregnancy cohort study followed for 14 years. *Journal of Pediatrics, 156*(4), 568-574.

Orr, S. T., Reiter, J.P., Blazer, D.G., & James, S.A. (2007). Maternal prenatal pregnancy-related anxiety and spontaneous preterm birth in Baltimore, Maryland. *Psychosomatic Medicine, 69*, 566-570.

Pace, T. W., Hu, F., & Miller, A. H. (2007). Cytokine-effects on glucocorticoid receptor function: Relevance to glucocorticoid resistance and the pathophysiology and treatment of major depression. *Brain, Behavior and Immunity, 21*(1), 9-19.

Parker, G., Gibson, N.A., Brotchie, H., Heruc, G., Rees, A-M., & Hadzi-Pavlovic, D. (2006). Omega-3 fatty acids and mood disorders. *American Journal of Psychiatry, 163*, 969-978.

Pasceri, V., Cheng, J. S., Willerson, J. T., & Yeh, E. T. (2001). Modulation of C-reactive protein-mediated monocyte chemoattractant protein-1 induction in human endothelial cells by anti-atherosclerosis drugs. *Circulation, 103*(21), 2531-2534.

Pasceri, V., Willerson, J. T., & Yeh, E. T. (2000). Direct proinflammatory effect of C-reactive protein on human endothelial cells. *Circulation, 102*(18), 2165-2168.

Pettersson-Kastberg, J., Mossberg, A. K., Trulsson, M., Yong, Y. J., Min, S., Lim, Y., et al. (2009). alpha-Lactalbumin, engineered to be nonnative and inactive, kills tumor cells when in complex with oleic acid. A new biological function resulting from partial unfolding. *Journal of Molecular Biology, 394*(5), 994-1010.

Pulkki-Raback, L., Elovainio, M., Kivimaki, M., Mattsson, N., Raitakari, O. T., Puttonen, S., et al. (2009). Depressive symptoms and the metabolic syndrome in childhood and adulthood: A prospective cohort study. *Health Psychology, 28*(1), 108-116.

Qiu, Y., Bevan, H., Weeraperuma, S., Wratting, D., Murphy, D., Neal, C. R., et al. (2008). Mammary alveolar development during lactation is inhibited by the endogenous antiangiogenic growth factor isoform, VEGF165b. The *FASEB Journal, 22*(4), 1104-1112.

Quillin, S. I. M., & Glenn, L. L. (2004). Interaction between feeding method and co-sleeping on maternal-newborn sleep. *Journal of Obstetric, Gynecologic and Neonatal Nursing, 33*(5), 580-588.

Qureshi, G. A., Hansen, S., & Sodersten, P. (1987). Offspring control of cerebrospinal fluid GABA concentrations in lactating rats. *Neuroscience Letters, 75*(1), 85-88.

Raghupathy, R., & Kalinka, J. (2008). Cytokine imbalance in pregnancy complications and its modulation. *Frontiers in Bioscience, 13*, 985-994.

Raikkonen, K., Matthews, K. A., & Salomon, K. (2003). Hostility predicts metabolic syndrome risk factors in children and adolescents. *Health Psychology, 22*, 279-286.

Ram, K. T., Bobby, P., Hailpern, S. M., Lo, J. C., Schocken, M., Skurnick, J., & Santoro, N. (2008). Duration of lactation is associated with lower prevalence of the metabolic syndrome in midlife--SWAN, the study of women's health across the nation. *American Journal of Obstetrics and Gynecology, 198*(3), e1-6.

Ranjit, N., Diez-Roux, A.V., Shea, S., Cushman, M., Seeman, T., Jackson, S.A., & Ni, H. (2007). Psychosocial factors and inflammation in the Multi-Ethnic Study of Atherosclerosis. *Archives of Internal Medicine, 167*, 174-181.

Rasmussen, K. M., & Kjolhede, C. L. (2004). Prepregnant overweight and obesity diminish the prolactin response to suckling in the first week postpartum. *Pediatrics, 113*(5), e465-471.

Redwine, L. S., Altemus, M., Leong, Y. M., & Carter, C. S. (2001). Lymphocyte responses to stress in postpartum women: Relationship to vagal tone. *Psychoneuroendocrinology, 26*(3), 241-251.

Rees, A. M., Austin, M. P., & Parker, G. (2005). Role of omega-3 fatty acids as a treatment for depression in the perinatal period. *Australia & New Zealand Journal of Psychiatry, 39*, 274-280.

Rieckmann, N., Gerin, W., Kronish, I. M., Burg, M. M., Chaplin, W. F., Kong, G., et al. (2006). Course of depressive symptoms and medication adherence after acute coronary syndromes: an electronic medication monitoring study. *Journal of the American College of Cardiology, 48*(11), 2218-2222.

Righard, L., & Alade, M. O. (1990). Effect of delivery room routines on success of first breast-feed. *Lancet, 336*(8723), 1105-1107.

Robles, T. F., Glaser, R., & Kiecolt-Glaser, J. K. (2005). Out of balance: A new look at chronic stress, depression, and immunity. *Current Directions in Psychological Science, 14*, 111-115.

Rohde, P., Ichikawa, L., Simon, G. E., Ludman, E. J., Linde, J. A., Jeffery, R. W., & Operskalski, B. H. (2008). Associations of child sexual and physical abuse with obesity and depression in middle-aged women. *Child Abuse & Neglect, 32*(9), 878-887.

Rosenman, R. H., & Friedman, M. (1974). Neurogenic factors in pathogenesis of coronary heart disease. *Medical Clinics of North America, 58*(2), 269-279.

Rosenspire, A. J., Kindzelskii, A. L., & Petty, H. R. (2002). Cutting edge: fever-associated temperatures enhance neutrophil responses to lipopolysaccharide: a potential mechanism involving cell metabolism. *Journal of Immunology, 169*(10), 5396-5400.

Roumestan, C., Michel, A., Bichon, F., Portet, K., Detoc, M., Henriquet, C., et al. (2007). Anti-inflammatory properties of desipramine and fluoxetine. *Respiratory Research, 8*, 35.

Rupke, S. J., Blecke, D., & Renfrow, M. (2006). Cognitive therapy for depression. *American Family Physician, 73*, 83-86.

Russo, J., Balogh, G. A., Chen, J., Fernandez, S. V., Fernbaugh, R., Heulings, R., et al. (2006). The concept of stem cell in the mammary gland and its implication in morphogenesis, cancer and prevention. *Frontiers in Bioscience, 11*, 151-172.

Rusterholz, C., Hahn, S., & Holzgreve, W. (2007). Role of placentally produced inflammatory and regulatory cytokines in pregnancy and the etiology of preeclampsia. *Seminars in Immunopathology, 29*(2), 151-162.

Rutledge, T., Reis, S. E., Olson, M., Owens, J., Kelsey, S. F., Pepine, C. J., et al. (2006). Depression is associated with cardiac symptoms, mortality risk, and hospitalization among women with suspected coronary disease: the NHLBI-sponsored WISE study. *Psychosomatic Medicine, 68*(2), 217-223. doi: 68/2/217 [pii]

Sabbaj, S., Ghosh, M. K., Edwards, B. H., Leeth, R., Decker, W. D., Goepfert, P. A., et al. (2005). Breast milk-derived antigen-specific CD8+ T cells: an extralymphoid effector memory cell population in humans. *Journal of Immunology, 174*(5), 2951-2956.

Sareen, J., Cox, B. J., Stein, M. B., Afifi, T. O., Fleet, C., & Asmundson, G. J. (2007). Physical and mental comorbidity, disability, and suicidal behavior associated with posttraumatic stress disorder in a large community sample. *Psychosomatic Medicine, 69*(3), 242-248.

Schuder, S. (2005). Stress-induced hypocortisolemia diagnosed as psychiatric disorders responsive to hypdrocortisone replacement. *Annals of the New York Academy of Sciences, 1057*, 466-478.

Schwarz, E. B., McClure, C. K., Tepper, P. G., Thurston, R., Janssen, I., Matthews, K. A., et al. (2010). Lactation and maternal measures of subclinical cardiovascular disease. *Obstetrics and Gynecology, 115*(1), 41-48.

Schwarz, E. B., Ray, R. M., Stuebe, A. M., Allison, M. A., Ness, R. B., Freiberg, M. S., et al. (2009). Duration of lactation and risk factors for maternal cardiovascular disease. *Obstetrics and Gynecology, 113*(5), 974-982.

Selye, H. (1956). Endocrine reactions during stress. *Current Research in Anesthesia and Analgesia, 35*(3), 182-193.

Shanks, N., Kusnecov, A., Pezzone, M., Berkun, J., & Rabin, B. S. (1997). Lactation alters the effects of conditioned stress on immune function. *American Journal of Physiology, 272*(1 Pt 2), R16-25.

Shizuya, K., Komori, T., Fujiwara, R., Miyahara, S., Ohmori, M., & Nomura, J. (1997). The influence of restraint stress on the expression of mRNAs for IL-6 and the IL-6 receptor in the hypothalamus and midbrain of the rat. *Life Science, 61*, 135-140.

Shizuya, K., Komori, T., Fujiwara, R., Miyahara, S., Ohmori, M., & Nomura, J. (1998). The expressions of mRNAs for interleukin-6 (IL-6) and the IL-6 receptor (IL-6R) in the rat hypothalamus and midbrain during restraint stress. *Life Science, 62*, 2315-2320.

Sibolboro Mezzacappa, E., & Endicott, J. (2007). Parity mediates the association between infant feeding method and maternal depressive symptoms in the postpartum. *Archives of Womens Mental Health, 10*(6), 259-266.

Slattery, D. A., & Neumann, I. D. (2010). Chronic icv oxytocin attenuates the pathological high anxiety state of selectively bred Wistar rats. *Neuropharmacology, 58*(1), 56-61.

Slopen, N., Lewis, T. T., Gruenewald, T. L., Mujahid, M. S., Ryff, C. D., Albert, M. A., & Williams, D. R. (2010). Early life adversity and inflammation in African Americans and whites in midlife in the United States Survey. *Psychosomatic Medicine, 72*, 694-701.

Smith, T. W. (1992). Hostility and health: Current status of a psychosomatic hypothesis. *Health Psychology, 11*, 139-150.

Smith, T. W., & Ruiz, J. M. (2002). Psychosocial influences on the development and course of coronary heart disease: Current status and implications for research and practice. *Journal of Consulting and Clinical Psychology, 70*, 548-568.

Smith, R., Chan, E. C., Bowman, M. E., Harewood, W. J., & Phippard, A. F. (1993). Corticotropin-releasing hormone in baboon pregnancy. *Journal of Clinical Endocrinology and Metabolism, 76*(4), 1063-1068.

Smith, T. W., Uchino, B. N., Berg, C. A., Florsheim, P., Pearce, G., Hawkins, M., et al. (2007). Hostile personality traits and coronary artery calcification in middle-aged and older married couples: Different effects for self-reports versus spouse ratings. *Psychosomatic Medicine, 69,* 441-448.

Spitzer, C., Barnow, S., Volzke, H., Wallaschotski, H., John, U., Freyberger, H. J., et al. (2010). Association of posttraumatic stress disorder with low-grade elevation of C-reactive protein: Evidence from the general population. *Journal of Psychiatric Research, 44*(1), 15-21.

Starkweather, A. R. (2007). The effects of exercise on perceived stress and IL-6 levels among older adults. *Biological Research for Nursing, 8,* 1-9.

Stein, M. B., Belik, S. L., Jacobi, F., & Sareen, J. (2008). Impairment associated with sleep problems in the community: Relationship to physical and mental health comorbidity. *Psychosomatic Medicine, 70,* 913-919.

Steptoe, A., Willemsen, G., Owen, N., Flower, L., & Mohamed-Ali, V. (2001). Acute mental stress elicits delayed increases in circulating inflammatory cytokine levels. *Clinical Sciences, 101,* 185-192.

Sternberg, E. M. (2006). Neural regulation of innate immunity: a coordinated nonspecific host response to pathogens. *Nature Reviews: Immunology, 6*(4), 318-328.

Stewart, J. C., Janicki-Deverts, D., Muldoon, M. F., & Kamarck, T. W. (2008). Depressive symptoms moderate the influence of hostility on serum Interleukin-6 and C-reactive protein. *Psychosomatic Medicine, 70,* 197-204.

Stock, S., & Uvnas-Moberg, K. (1988). Increased plasma levels of oxytocin in response to afferent electrical stimulation of the sciatic and vagal nerves and in response to touch and pinch in anaesthetized rats. *Acta Physiologica Scandinavica, 132*(1), 29-34.

Strathearn, L., Mamun, A. A., Najman, J. M., & O'Callaghan, M. J. (2009). Does breastfeeding protect against substantiated child abuse and neglect? A 15-year cohort study. *Pediatrics, 123*(2), 483-493.

Stuebe, A. M., Rich-Edwards, J. W., Willett, W. C., Manson, J. E., & Michels, K. B. (2005). Duration of lactation and incidence of type-2 diabetes. *Journal of the American Medical Association, 294*(20), 2601-2610.

Stuebe, A. M., & Rich-Edwards, J. W. (2009). The reset hypothesis: Lactation and maternal metabolism. *American Journal of Perinatology, 26*(1), 81-88.

Su, K. P. (2009). Biological mechanisms of antidepressant effect of Omega-3 fatty acids: How does fish oil act as a "mind-body interface"? *Neurosignal, 17,* 144-152.

Suarez, E. C. (2003). Joint effect of hostility and severity of depressive symptoms on plasma Interleukin-6 concentration. *Psychosomatic Medicine, 65*, 523-527.

Suarez, E. C. (2006). Sex differences in the relation of depressive symptoms, hostility, and anger expression to indices of glucose metabolism in nondiabetic adults. *Health Psychology, 25*, 484-492.

Suarez, E. C., & Goforth, H. (2010). Sleep and inflammation: A potential link to chronic diseases. In K. A. Kendall-Tackett (Ed.), *The psychoneuroimmunology of chronic disease* (pp. 53-75). Washington, DC: American Psychological Association.

Suarez, E. C., Lewis, J. G., Krishnan, R. R., & Young, K. H. (2004). Enhanced expression of cytokines and chemokines by blood monocytes to in vitro lipopolysaccharide stimulation are associated with hostility and severity of depressive symptoms in healthy women. *Psychoneuroendocrinology, 29*, 1119-1128.

Sun, B., Fujiwara, K., Adachi, S., & Inoue, K. (2005). Physiological roles of prolactin-releasing peptide. *Regulatory Peptides, 126*(1-2), 27-33.

Surtees, P., Wainwright, N., Day, N., Brayne, C., Luben, R., & Khaw, K. T. (2003). Adverse experience in childhood as a developmental risk factor for altered immune status in adulthood. *International Journal of Behavioral Medicine, 10*(3), 251-268.

Szelenyi, J., & Vizi, E. S. (2007). The catecholamine cytokine balance: interaction between the brain and the immune system. *Annals of the New York Academy of Science, 1113*, 311-324. 10.1196/annals.1391.026

Taylor, C. B., Conrad, A., Wilhelm, F. H., Neri, E., DeLorenzo, A., Kramer, M. A., et al. (2006). Psychophysiological and cortisol responses to psychological stress in depressed and nondepressed older men and women with elevated cardiovascular disease risk. *Psychosomatic Medicine, 68*(4), 538-546.

Teegen, F. (1999). Childhood sexual abuse and long-term sequelae. In A. Maercker, M. Schutzwohl & Z. Solomon (Eds.), *Posttraumatic stress disorder: A lifespan developmental perspective* (pp. 97-112). Seattle: Hogrefe & Huber.

Thayer, J., & Sternberg, E. (2006). Beyond heart rate variability: Vagal regulation of allostatic systems. *Annals of the New York Academy of Sciences, 1088*, 361-372.

Thornton, L. M., Andersen, B. L., Schuler, T. A., & Carson, W. E. R. (2009). A psychological intervention reduces inflammatory markers by alleviating depresseive symptoms: Secondard analysis of a randomized controlled trial. *Psychosomatic Medicine, 71*(7), 715-724.

Toufexis, D. J., & Walker, C. D. (1996). Noradrenergic facilitation of the adrenocorticotropin response to stress is absent during lactation in the rat. *Brain Research, 737*(1-2), 71-77.

Tsigos, C., & Chrousos, G. P. (2002). Hypothalamic-pituitary-adrenal axis, neuroendocrine factors and stress. *Journal of Psychosomatic Research, 53*, 865-871.

Udall, J. N., Jr. (2007). Infant feeding: initiation, problems, approaches. *Current Problems in Pediatric and Adolescent Health Care, 37*(10), 374-399.

Uvnas-Moberg, K. (1997). Physiological and endocrine effects of social contact. *Annals of the New York Academy of Sciences, 807*, 146-163.

Vaccarino, V., McClure, C., Johnson, D., Sheps, D. S., Bittner, V., Rutledge, T., Merz, C. N. B. (2008). Depression, the metabolic syndrome and cardiovascular risk. *Psychosomatic Medicine, 70*, 40-48.

Valham, F., Stegmayr, B., Eriksson, M., Hagg, E., Lindberg, E., & Franklin, K. A. (2009). Snoring and witnessed sleep apnea is related to diabetes mellitus in women. *Sleep Medicine, 10*, 112-117.

Vollmar, P., Haghikia, A., Dermietzel, R., & Faustmann, P. M. (2007). Venlafaxine exhibits an anti-inflammatory effect in an inflammatory co-culture model. *International Journal of Neuropsychopharmacology*, 2008 Feb;11(1):111-7.

von Kanel, R., Hepp, U., Buddeberg, C., Keel, M., Mica, L., Aschbacher, K., & Schnyder, U. (2006). Altered blood coagulation in patients with posttraumatic stress disorder. *Psychosomatic Medicine, 68*(4), 598-604.

Walters, M. W., Boggs, K. M., Ludington-Hoe, S., Price, K. M., & Morrison, B. (2007). Kangaroo care at birth for full term infants: a pilot study. *MCN American Journal of Maternal Child Nursing, 32*(6), 375-381.

Wang, C., Chung, M., Lichtenstein, A., Balk, E., Kupelnick, B., DeVine, D., et al. (2004). Effects of omega-3 fatty acids on cardiovascular disease (Vol. AHRQ Publication No. 04-E009-1). Rockville, MD: Agency for Healthcare Research and Quality.

Warner, R., Appleby, L., Whitton, A., & Faragher, B. (1996). Demographic and obstetric risk factors for postnatal psychiatric morbidity. *British Journal of Psychiatry, 168*(5), 607-611.

Watkins, L. R., & Maier, S. F. (2000). The pain of being sick: Implications of immune-to-brain communication for understanding pain. *Annual Review of Psychology, 51*, 29-57.

Werneke, U., Turner, T., & Priebe, S. (2006). Complementary medicines in psychiatry: Review of effectiveness and safety. *British Journal of Psychiatry, 188*, 109-121.

Williams, M. J., Williams, S. M., & Poulton, R. (2006). Breast feeding is related to C reactive protein concentration in adult women. *Journal of Epidemiology and Community Health, 60*, 146-148.

Wilson, C. J., Finch, C.E., & Cohen, H.J. (2002). Cytokines and cognition—The case for a head-to-toe inflammatory paradigm. *Journal of the American Geriatrics Society, 50*, 2041-2056.

Wilson, A. M., Ryan, M. C., & Boyle, A. J. (2006). The novel role of C-reactive protein in cardiovascular disease: risk marker or pathogen. *International Journal of Cardiology, 106*(3), 291-297.

Windle, R. J., Brady, M. M., Kunanandam, T., Da Costa, A. P., Wilson, B. C., Harbuz, M., et al. (1997). Reduced response of the hypothalamo-pituitary-adrenal axis to alpha1 agonist stimulation during lactation. *Endocrinology, 138*(9), 3741-3748.

Wong, A.W., & Rosh, A.J. (2010). Postpartum infections. Retrieved March 8, 2011, from http://emedicine.medscape.com/article/796892-overview.

Woods, A. B., Page, G. G., O'Campo, P., Pugh, L. C., Ford, D., & Campbell, J. C. (2005). The mediation effect of posttraumatic stress disorder symptoms on the relationship of intimate partner violence and IFN-gamma levels. *American Journal of Community Psychology, 36*(1-2), 159-175. doi: 10.1007/s10464-005-6240-7

Wurglics, M., & Schubert-Zsilavecz, M. (2006). Hypericum perforatum: A "modern" herbal antidepressant: Pharmacokinetics of active ingredients. *Clinical Pharmacokinetics, 45*, 449-468.

Wust, S., Federenko, I., Hellhammer, D., & Kirschbaum, C. (2000). Genetic factors, perceived chronic stress, and the free cortisol response to awakening. *Psychoneuroendocrinology, 25*, 707-720.

Yehuda, R. (1997). Sensitization of the hypothalamic-pituitary-adrenal axis in posttraumatic stress disorder. *Annals of the New York Academy of Sciences, 821*, 57-75.

Zanoli, P. (2004). Role of hyperforin in the pharmacological activities of St. John's wort. *CNS, 10*, 203-218. not in Pubmed

Zheng, T., Duan, L., Liu, Y., Zhang, B., Wang, Y., Chen, Y., et al. (2000). Lactation reduces breast cancer risk in Shandong Province, China. *American Journal of Epidemiology, 152*(12), 1129-1135.

Zhou, C., Tabb, M.M., Sadatrafiei, A., Grun, F., Sun, A., & Blumberg, B. (2004). Hyperforin, the active component of St. John's wort, induces IL-8 expression in human intestinal epithelial cells via a MAPK-dependent, NF-kappaB-independent pathway. *Journal of Clinical Immunology, 24*, 623-636.

Zouridakis, E., Avanzas, P., Arroyo-Espliguero, R., Fredericks, S., & Kaski, J. C. (2004). Markers of inflammation and rapid coronary artery disease progression in patients with stable angina pectoris. *Circulation, 110*(13), 1747-1753.

Zwaka, T. P., Hombach, V., & Torzewski, J. (2001). C-reactive protein-mediated low density lipoprotein uptake by macrophages: Implications for atherosclerosis. *Circulation, 103*(9), 1194-1197.

Index

Author Bios

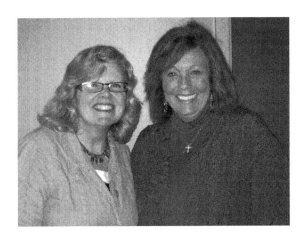

Maureen Groer, RN, PhD, FAAN

Maureen Groer is a family nurse practitioner and has a PhD in human physiology. Her work has focused on understanding stress and health in women and infants through the lens of psychoneuroimmunology. She currently runs a large and productive Biobehavioral laboratory at the University of South Florida, College of Nursing in Tampa, Florida, where she holds the Gordon Keller Endowed professorship. She has written three textbooks in Pathophysiology, and has authored over 50 research papers in refereed journals. Dr. Groer has been funded by the National Institutes of Health since 2001 to study the influence of lactation on postpartum stress and immunity. Dr. Groer teaches pathophysiology and philosophy of science to graduate students and breastfeeding to undergraduate students.

Kathleen Kendall-Tackett, Ph.D., IBCLC, FAPA

Dr. Kendall-Tackett is a health psychologist and an International Board Certified Lactation Consultant. She is a Clinical Associate Professor of Pediatrics at Texas Tech University School of Medicine in Amarillo, Texas, and a Fellow of the American Psychological Association in both the Divisions of Health and Trauma Psychology. Dr. Kendall-Tackett is Associate Editor of the journal *Psychological Trauma,* and editor-in-chief of *Clinical Lactation.* Dr. Kendall-Tackett is author of more than 280 journal articles, book chapters and other publications, and author or editor of 21 books in the fields of trauma, women's health, depression, and breastfeeding. She is a founding officer of the American Psychological Association's Division of Trauma Psychology, and is currently serving her second term as Division Secretary.

Ordering Information

Hale Publishing, L.P.

1712 N. Forest Street

Amarillo, Texas, USA 79106

8:00 am to 5:00 pm CST

Call » 806.376.9900

Toll free » 800.378.1317

Fax » 806.376.9901

Online Orders

www.ibreastfeeding.com